Mneumonic for resuscitation

O – oxygen
W – weight
E – electricity (Joules)
T – tracheal tube (ETT)
F – fluids
A – adrenaline
G – glucose

Weight (kg) over 1 yr =
(age yrs + 4) × 2

ETT size (mm) over 1 yr =
(age yrs ÷ 4) + 4

SAFE APPROACH
S – shout for help
A – approach with care
F – free from danger
E – evaluate ABC

Systolic BP guide (mmHg) =
(age yrs ×2) + 80

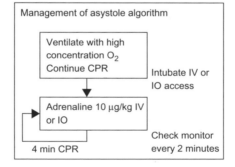

Management of asystole algorithm

Ventilate with high
concentration O_2
Continue CPR

Intubate IV or
IO access

Adrenaline 10 µg/kg IV
or IO

4 min CPR

Check monitor
every 2 minutes

For Mary Pow. . . . a shining light in life,
and for Andy and Izzy with love, JD

For Martin and Cherry Hassell,
with love, LLH

For Elsevier:
Senior Commissioning Editor: Ninette Premdas
Project Development Manager: Katrina Mather, Gill Cloke
Project Manager: Christine Johnston
Design: Keith Kail
Illustrator: David Gardner, Annabel Milne
Illustration Manager: Gillian Richards
Photographer (cover photo): Piers Allardyce

Children in Intensive Care

A Survival Guide

SECOND EDITION

Joanna H Davies BSc (Hons) RGN RSCN ENB 415
Sister and Retrieval Nurse Practitioner, Paediatric Intensive Care,
Evelina Children's Hospital, St Thomas' Hospital, Guy's and St Thomas'
NHS Foundation Trust, London, UK

Lynda L Hassell BSc (Hons), MSc RGN RSCN ENB 415
Head of Nursing, Paediatrics, St Mary's NHS Trust, London, UK

Foreword by

Ian Murdoch BSc MBBS DCH FRCP
Director of Paediatric Intensive Care, Evelina Children's Hospital,
St Thomas' Hospital, Guy's and St Thomas' NHS Foundation Trust,
London, UK

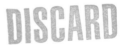

CHURCHILL
LIVINGSTONE

ELSEVIER

Edinburgh   London   New York   Oxford   Philadelphia   St Louis   Sydney   Toronto   2007

CHURCHILL
LIVINGSTONE
ELSEVIER

An imprint of Elsevier Limited

© Harcourt Publishers Limited 2001
© 2007, Elsevier Limited. All rights reserved.

The right of Joanna H Davies and Lynda L Hassell to be identified as authors of this work
has been asserted by them in accordance with the Copyright, Designs and Patents Act 1988

First edition 2001
Second edition 2007

ISBN-13: 978 0 443 10023 9

British Library Cataloguing in Publication Data
A catalogue record for this book is available from the British Library

Library of Congress Cataloging in Publication Data
A catalog record for this book is available from the Library of Congress

Note
Knowledge and best practice in this field are constantly changing. As new research and
experience broaden our knowledge, changes in practice, treatment and drug therapy may
become necessary or appropriate. Readers are advised to check the most current information
provided (i) on procedures featured or (ii) by the manufacturer of each product to be
administered, to verify the recommended dose or formula, the method and duration of
administration, and contraindications. It is the responsibility of the practitioner, relying on
their own experience and knowledge of the patient, to make diagnoses, to determine dosages
and the best treatment for each individual patient, and to take all appropriate safety
precautions. To the fullest extent of the law, neither the Publisher nor the Authors assume any
liability for any injury and/or damage to persons or property arising out or related to any use
of the material contained in this book.

The Publisher

The
Publisher's
policy is to use
**paper manufactured
from sustainable forests**

Printed in China

CONTENTS

FOREWORD

The delivery of paediatric intensive care in the UK has grown significantly over the last decade. The overwhelming majority of critically ill children are now managed in dedicated paediatric intensive care units staffed by highly skilled and trained medical and nursing professionals. Introduction of the Intensive Care Nursing of Children course (ENB 415) in the 1980s led to the development of other higher educational programmes such as the BSc in Nursing with paediatric critical care as the focus. Today there are many postgraduate courses for nurses to further gain advanced nursing skills in this growing field. However, putting theory into practice frequently leaves the intensive care clinician, be it doctor, nurse or paramedic, in a daunting situation that demands a wide, extensive knowledge of medicine at one's fingertips. The aim of this manual is to fill that gap.

This manual offers a wealth of accessible information for newcomers to paediatric intensive care and old timers alike. The emphasis is on the simple and practical. It is a concise and comprehensive reference manual for use in wards, theatres or on retrieval, and covers a wide range of topics from anatomy and physiology to drug therapy and X-ray interpretation. This is the second update of a successful recipe, where the simple layout combines essential information with graphs, tables and informative references without losing clarity. Useful information on practical issues that frequently occur in the intensive care setting, such as drug dosages, drug compatibility lists and reference ranges, are also provided that are hard to find in many of the larger critical care reference books. As well as introducing a host of new topics such as non-invasive ventilation and capnography, this book offers broad management guidelines and treatment algorithms for common intensive care problems. It is not a replacement for the well tested and fine-tuned protocols that many established units have developed over the years but a framework for where none exist. It is hoped, in addition to its role as a bedside learning tool, that this pocket book makes the difficult task of caring for the critically ill child that little bit easier.

Ian Murdoch
Director of Paediatric Intensive Care
St Thomas' Hospital,
Guy's and St Thomas' NHS Foundation Trust,
London

PREFACE

The concept of this book began in the notepads of paediatric intensive care nurses, who care for critically ill children with a huge variety of conditions including complex cardiac defects, bronchiolitis, meningococcal septicaemia and specific metabolic disorders. It was evident that a quick point of reference was required that outlined handy hints for emergency situations and gave practical tips for coping with acutely ill children and troubleshooting technical equipment, together with normal values and drug equations. This is not intended as a textbook but aims to complement such books by providing instant access to concise, valuable nuggets of information that we hope will stimulate a desire to seek out more in-depth knowledge.

The second edition of this book has been edited to incorporate readers' feedback while maintaining its pocket size. This has included the revision of all chapters and the addition of new information. For example, we have added a quick guide for interpretation of chest X-rays, information on non-invasive ventilation and capnography, a new chapter on child protection issues and the new immunisation schedule, as well as updating resuscitation guidelines. This quick reference guide is intended for all those who come into contact with critically ill and high-dependency children in accident and emergency departments, general paediatric wards, high-dependency units, theatres and adult and paediatric intensive care units.

We have tried to select data that we have found particularly useful on a day-to-day basis and amalgamated it into a portable format. We have endeavoured to provide concise and up-to-date information but, as treatments and drug doses change rapidly, please also consult local policies, paediatric formularies and current research.

London, 2007

Jo Davies
Lynda Hassell

ACKNOWLEDGEMENTS

The authors wish to thank and acknowledge the help, advice and support of the following people:

Sally Adams	Senior Paediatric Physiotherapist, Evelina Children's Hospital
Sara Arenas Lopez	Senior Paediatric Pharmacist, PICU, Evelina Children's Hospital
Carmen Barton	Lead Nurse Paediatric Nephrology, Evelina Children's Hospital
Fiona Bickell	Regional Retrieval Co-ordinator, South Thames Region
Mark Clement	Nurse Practitioner, Children's Acute Transport Service
Mollie Cook	Nurse Counsellor, Paediatrics, Evelina Children's Hospital
Mehrengise Cooper	Consultant in PICU, St Mary's NHS Trust
Helen Day	Paediatric Critical Care Educator, Kings College Hospital
Sasha Herring	Sister, PICU, Evelina Children's Hospital
Frances Court Brown	Paediatric Dietician, Evelina Children's Hospital
Mike Champion	Paediatric Metabolic Consultant, Evelina Children's Hospital
Andrew Durward	Consultant Paediatric Intensivist, Evelina Children's Hospital
Jane Gick	Paediatric Metabolic Nurse Specialist, St Mary's NHS Trust
Jo Hand	Metabolic Dietician, St Mary's NHS Trust
Judith Harris	Lecturer Practitioner, Evelina Children's Hospital
Clare Harrison	Consultant Haematologist, Guy's & St Thomas' NHS Foundation Trust
Kelly Larmour	Paediatric Dietician, Evelina Children's Hospital
Fiona Lynch	Sister, PICU, Evelina Children's Hospital
Rosan Meyer	Paediatric Research Dietician, Imperial College
Ian Murdoch	Director of PICU, Evelina Children's Hospital

John Richardson – Donor Transplant Co-ordinator, South Thames Transplant Co-ordination Service

Shelley Riphagen – Consultant Paediatric Intensivist, Evelina Children's Hospital

Steve Tomlin – Senior Paediatric Pharmacist, Evelina Children's Hospital

Robert Urquhart – Senior Paediatric Pharmacist, The Royal Free Hospital

Carol Williams – Nurse Consultant, PICU, Evelina Children's Hospital

Edward Koa Wing – Chief Medical Technologist (Retired) Guy's & St Thomas' NHS Foundation Trust

We also wish to thank our friends and colleagues in PICU at both Evelina Children's Hospital and St Mary's Hospital, London.

ABBREVIATIONS

ABC	Airway, breathing, circulation	COHb	Carboxyhaemoglobin
ABG	Arterial blood gas	CPAP	Continuous positive airways pressure
ACT	Activated clotting time	CPB	Cardiopulmonary bypass
ADH	Antidiuretic hormone	CPDA	Added citrate, phosphate, dextrose and adenine
A&E	Accident and Emergency		
AED	Automated external defibrillator	CPP	Cerebral perfusion pressure
ALP	Alkaline phosphatase	CPR	Cardiopulmonary resuscitation
ALT	Alanine transaminase		
APTT	Activated prothrombin time	CSF	Cerebrospinal fluid
		CT	Computed tomography
ARDS	Adult respiratory distress syndrome	CVP	Central venous pressure
		CVVH	Continuous veno-venous haemofiltration
ARF	Acute renal failure		
ASD	Atrial septal defect	CVVHD	Continuous veno-venous haemodiafiltration
AV	Atrioventricular		
AVSD	Atrioventricular septal defect	DC	Direct current
BFR	Blood flow rate	DDAVP	1-deamino 8-D arginine vasopressin
BP	Blood pressure		
bpm	Beats per minute	DIC	Disseminated intravascular coagulation
BSA	Body surface area		
BSE	Bovine spongiform encephalopathy		
		DKA	Diabetic ketoacidosis
cAMP	Cyclic adenosine monophosphate	DO_2	Oxygen delivery
		DORV	Double outlet right ventricle
CBF	Cerebral blood flow		
CBV	Cerebral blood volume	ECG	Electrocardiogram/ electrocardiography
CEN	European Committee for Standardisation		
		ECMO	Extracorporeal membrane oxygenation
CFAM	Cerebral function analysing monitor		
		EEG	Electroencephalogram/ electroencephalography
CMV	Controlled mandatory ventilation; cytomegalovirus		
		EMD	Electromechanical dissociation
CNS	Central nervous system	EMG	Electromyography
CO	Cardiac output	ESR	Erythrocyte sedimentation rate
CO_2	Carbon dioxide		

ET	Endotracheal	MAP	Mean airways pressure; mean systemic arterial pressure
ETT	Endotracheal tube		
FFP	Fresh frozen plasma		
F_iO_2	Fractional concentration of inspired oxygen	MCH	Mean corpuscular haemoglobin
		MCV	Mean corpuscular volume
FRC	Functional residual capacity	MMR	Measles, mumps and rubella
GCS	Glasgow Coma Scale		
GGT	Gamma–glutamyl transpeptidase	MRI	Magnetic resonance imaging
GTN	Glyceryl trinitrate	$NaHCO_3$	Sodium bicarbonate
H^+	Hydrogen ion	NG	Nasogastric
Hb	Haemoglobin	NO	Nitric oxide
HCO_3	Carbonic acid	NO_2	Nitrogen dioxide
HFO	High-frequency oscillation	O_2	Oxygen
		OH^-	Hydroxyl ion
HFOV	High-frequency oscillation ventilation	OLT	Orthoptic liver transplantation
Hib	*Haemophilus influenzae* type b	PA	Pulmonary artery
		P_aCO_2	Partial pressure of carbon dioxide in arterial blood
HIV	Human immuno-deficiency virus		
HLHS	Hypoplastic left heart syndrome	P_aO_2	Partial pressure of oxygen in arterial blood
HUS	Haemolytic–uraemic syndrome	PAP	Pulmonary arterial pressure
ICP	Intracranial pressure	PCO_2	Partial pressure of carbon dioxide
IHSS	Idiopathic hypertrophic subaortic stenosis		
		PO_2	Partial pressure of oxygen
IM	Intramuscular	PCV	Packed cell volume
INR	International normalised ratio	PD	Peritoneal dialysis
		PDA	Patent ductus arteriosus
IO	Intraosseus		
IT	Inspired time	PDEIII	Phosphodiesterase III
ITP	Immune thrombocytopenia purpura	PEA	Pulseless electrical activity
IV	Intravenous	PEEP	Positive end-expiratory pressure
IVC	Inferior vena cava		
JET	Junctional ectopic tachycardia	PFO	Patent foramen ovale
		PICU	Paediatric intensive care unit
LA	Left atrium/atrial		
LAP	Left atrial pressure	PIP	Peak inspiratory pressure
LDH	Lactate dehydrogenase		
LV	Left ventricle/ventricular	PS	Pulmonary stenosis
		PT	Prothrombin time

PTFE	Polytretrafluorethylene (Gore-Tex®)	SVR	Systemic vascular resistance
PTT	Partial thromboplastin time	SVT	Supraventricular tachycardia
PTV	Patient trigger ventilation	TAPVD	Total anomalous pulmonary venous drainage
PVR	Pulmonary vascular resistance	TBSA	Total body surface area
RA	Right atrium/atrial		
RAP	Right atrial pressure	TGA	Transposition of the great arteries
RBC	Red blood cells		
RSV	Respiratory syncytial virus	TMP	Transmembrane pressure
RV	Right ventricle/ ventricular	TPN	Total parenteral nutrition
RVOT	Right ventricular outflow tract	TR–GVHD	Transfusion-related graft versus host disease
SA	Sinoatrial		
SAGM	Added sodium chloride, adenine, glucose and mannitol	UFR	Ultrafiltration rate
		UKCC	United Kingdom Central Council
S_aO_2	Arterial saturation of oxygen	VC	Volume control
		VF	Ventricular fibrillation
SBE	Subacute bacterial endocarditis	VS	Volume support
SIADH	Syndrome of inappropriate antidiuretic hormone secretion	VSD	Ventricular septal defect
		VT	Ventricular tachycardia
SIMV	Synchronised intermittent mandatory ventilation	WBC	White blood count
		WPW	Wolff–Parkinson–White
SVC	Superior vena cava		

ALL ABOUT RESUSCITATION

1

Recognition and prompt treatment of cardiorespiratory deterioration in children is a vital aspect of paediatric nursing in any environment but is particularly pertinent to paediatric intensive care. The ABC method of assessment can be used and children should be frequently reassessed as their condition may rapidly alter.

CARDIOPULMONARY ASSESSMENT

A Airway
B Breathing
C Circulation.

Airway

- Assess patency
- Assess ability to maintain independently with positioning and suction, or
- Assess need for adjuncts, e.g. rigid airway or endotracheal tube.

Breathing

Assess rate of breathing, depth, chest movement, air entry, the work of breathing, use of accessory muscles, recession, nasal flaring, grunting, wheeze, stridor, colour of patient.

Circulation

- Assess heart rate, blood pressure, central and peripheral pulses, skin perfusion, colour, mottling, capillary refill time, temperature – central and peripheral.

See covers for normal ranges of heart rate, blood pressure and respiratory rates for each age group.

Pulse volume is related to pulse pressure, i.e. the difference between the systolic and diastolic pressure. When there is decreased cardiac output, the pulse pressure narrows and pulses become weak.

It is also helpful to note level of consciousness, position, pupil reaction, muscle tone, urine output.

A quick guide for normal systolic blood pressure in a child 1 year or above

Median systolic blood pressure in children over 1 year of age: 80 mmHg + (2 × age in years)

THE SAFE APPROACH TO BASIC LIFE SUPPORT AND LIFE SUPPORT ALGORITHMS (ADVANCED LIFE SUPPORT GROUP 2006)

S Shout for help
A Approach with care
F Free from danger
E Evaluate ABC.

Figures 1.1 and 1.2 represent algorithms that are recommended for basic and advanced life support in emergency situations. Figures 1.3 and 1.4 represent algorithms for use when a child presents with ventricular tachycardia and supraventricular tachycardia and Figure 1.5 is an algorithm for the management of hyperkalaemia. Table 1.1 provides guidelines for drug treatment for tachycardia.

Non-shockable rhythm (asystole/pulseless electrical activity) (Resuscitation Council (UK) 2005)

- Perform continuous CPR
- If bag/mask ventilating – use 15 chest compressions to 2 ventilations for all ages
- If patient intubated, use continuous chest compressions
- Compression rate 100/min
- Give adrenaline (epinephrine) 10 µg/kg every 3–5 min
- Consider and correct reversible causes (e.g. alkalising agents).

Shockable rhythm (VF/pulseless VT) (Resuscitation Council (UK) 2005)

- Give **shock** of 4 J/kg then immediately resume CPR starting with chest compressions, without reassessing rhythm or feeling for a pulse
- Continue CPR for 2 min
- Pause briefly to check monitor and if still VF/pulseless VT, give second **shock** at 4 J/kg
- Resume CPR immediately after second shock. Consider and correct reversible causes (4 Hs and 4 Ts)
- Continue CPR for 2 min

Fig 1.1 Paediatric basic life support – health-care professionals with a duty to respond (with permission from Resuscitation Council (UK) 2005)

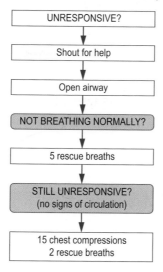

UNRESPONSIVE?

↓

Shout for help

↓

Open airway

↓

NOT BREATHING NORMALLY?

↓

5 rescue breaths

↓

STILL UNRESPONSIVE?
(no signs of circulation)

↓

15 chest compressions
2 rescue breaths

After 1 minute call resuscitation team then continue CPR.

 NB If there is any suspicion of trauma to the neck or spine, the neck and spine should be immobilised and the jaw thrust technique of opening the airway should be utilised.

The child should be approached correctly, gently stimulated for responsiveness and then treated using ABC.

The chest compression rate for all ages is 100/minute. In all children a ratio of 15 compressions to 2 ventilations should be used, but lone rescuers may use a ratio of 30:2, particularly if they are having difficulty with the transition between compression and ventilation.

Shockable rhythm (continued)

- Pause briefly to check monitor and if still VF/pulseless VT, give adrenaline (epinephrine) 10 μg/kg followed immediately by a third **shock** at 4 J/kg
- Resume CPR immediately for 2 min

Fig 1.2   Paediatric advanced life support (with permission from Resuscitation Council (UK) 2005)

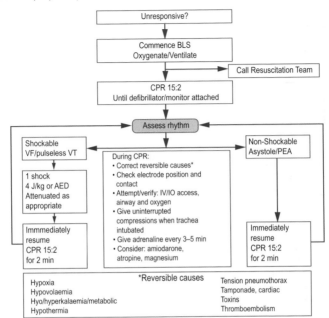

Shockable rhythm (continued)

- Pause briefly to check monitor and if still VF/pulseless VT, give IV bolus of amiodarone 5 mg/kg and an immediate fourth **shock**
- Continue with shocks every 2 min, minimising the breaks in chest compressions as much as possible
- Give adrenaline 10 µg/kg before every other shock until return of spontaneous circulation.

EARLY TREATMENT OF VENTRICULAR TACHYCARDIA (WITH PULSE) (ADVANCED LIFE SUPPORT GROUP 2006)

- Early consultation with paediatric cardiologist
- May suggest use of amiodarone or procainamide – both can cause hypotension, which should be treated with volume expansion
- Where VT has been caused by drug toxicity, sedation, and anaesthesia DC shock may be the safest approach – use synchronised shocks initially

Fig 1.3 Algorithm for the management of ventricular tachycardia (with permission from Advanced Life Support Group 2006)

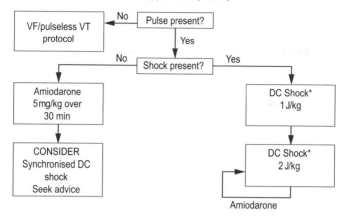

- as these are less likely to produce VF but, if they are ineffectual, subsequent attempts will have to be asynchronous if the child is in shock
- The treatment of torsades de pointes VT is magnesium sulphate by IV infusion (25–50 mg/kg (max. 2 g))
- Amiodarone 5 mg/kg may be given over a few minutes in VT if the child is in severe shock
- Seek advice.

PULSELESS ELECTRICAL ACTIVITY (PEA)

This was previously known as electromechanical dissociation or EMD.

There are recognisable complexes seen on the ECG monitor but there is an absence of palpable pulses and inadequate cardiac output.

Causes of PEA include four Hs and four Ts:

- Hypovolaemia (most common cause)
- Hypothermia
- Hypoxaemia
- Hyperkalaemia
- Tamponade
- Tension pneumothorax
- Thromboembolism
- Toxicity – i.e. drug overdose (commonly tricyclic antidepressants).

The underlying cause of PEA must be sought but PEA should be treated and managed like asystole until the specific cause has been identified and treated.

Fig 1.4 Algorithm for the management of supraventricular tachycardia (with permission from Advanced Life Support Group 2006)

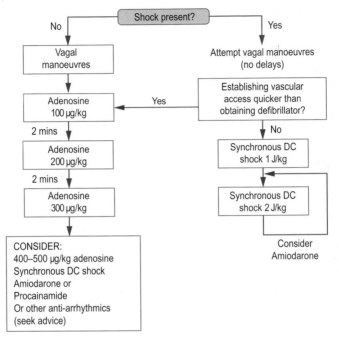

Resuscitation drug doses – cardiac arrest

- Adrenaline (epinephrine) 10 µg/kg (0.1 ml/kg of 1:10 000) via IV or IO route (maximum dose is 10 ml of 1:10 000)

  Subsequent doses of adrenaline will be the same and should be given every 3–5 min. The use of a higher dose of adrenaline via the IV or IO route is not recommended routinely in children. High-dose adrenaline has not been shown to improve survival or neurological outcome after cardiopulmonary arrest (Resuscitation Council (UK) 2005)

  Adrenaline can be given via the tracheal tube route at ten times the IV dose (100 µg/kg) but this route should be avoided if at all possible as evidence shows there may be a paradoxical effect (Resuscitation Council (UK) 2005)

- Sodium bicarbonate 8.4% 1 ml/kg

  This may be indicated if profound acidosis persists during an arrest situation but beware as this will increase intracellular carbon dioxide

Fig 1.5 Algorithm for the management of hyperkalaemia (with permission from Advanced Life Support Group 2006)

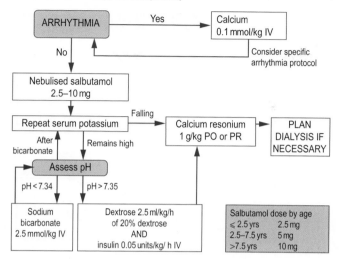

Hyperkalaemia (serum K + > 5.5 mmols/L) is a dangerous condition which may cause arrhythmias or death. It is most commonly caused by renal failure but may also be caused by potassium overload, loss of potassium from cells due to acidosis or celllysis, hypoaldosteronism and hypoadrenalism. If potassium is very high, more than one treatment can be used simultaneously.

levels so the patient should be receiving assisted ventilation. Sodium bicarbonate is also recommended in the treatment of hyperkalaemia and tricyclic antidepressant overdose

 Sodium bicarbonate inactivates adrenaline and dopamine so the IV line should be flushed well after use. Bicarbonate cannot be given via the endotracheal route. Bicarbonate cannot be given via the same IV line as calcium as precipitation will occur (Advanced Life Support Group 2006).

- **Atropine** 20 µg/kg (minimum dose 100 µg to prevent paradoxical bradycardia and maximum dose of 600 µg) is no longer recommended except in a patient who has developed bradycardia from vagal stimulation

Table 1.1 Guidelines for the drug treatment of tachycardia

The following are only guidelines as to the initial treatment of a specific arrhythmia; expert advice should be sought before prescribing or if there is a lack of response.

Arrhythmia	Initial treatment
Supraventricular tachycardia	1. Adenosine – repeat bolus when necessary 2. Digoxin 3. Propranolol 4. Flecainide 5. Verapamil
Sinus tachycardia	Find and treat underlying cause
Atrial fibrillation	1. Digoxin
Atrial flutter	2. Propranolol
Atrial tachycardia	3. Amiodarone
Ventricular tachycardia	1. Amiodarone 2. Lidocaine (lignocaine) (if no access or only drug available) 3. Magnesium sulphate
Wolff–Parkinson–White syndrome with atrial fibrillation	Amiodarone **Do not give digoxin or verapamil**

Source: with permission from Guy's, St Thomas', King's College and University Lewisham Hospitals 2005.

- **Calcium** is no longer recommended in the treatment of electro-mechanical dissociation and asystole. However it is indicated in documented hypocalcaemias, in hyperkalaemia and in the treatment of hypermagnesaemia and calcium channel overdose.

Emergency anti-arrhythmic drugs

- Amiodarone 5 mg/kg diluted to 4 ml/kg with 5% dextrose given over 30 min, IV or IO for shock-resistant ventricular fibrillation and pulse-less ventricular tachycardia (VF/VT). Use central vein if access available or a large peripheral vein (Advanced Life Support Group 2006)
- Adenosine Initially 100 µg/kg then 200 µg/kg, then 300 µg/kg up to a maximum dose of 500 µg/kg (300 µg/kg under 1 month of age) (Advanced Life Support Group 2006)
  Adenosine should be given as a fast IV bolus through a large peripheral or a central vein and followed immediately by a rapid saline flush for the treatment of supraventricular tachycardia resistant to vagal manoeuvres in patients who are not in shock (Advanced Life Support Group 2006). If the patient is in shock, then synchronised cardioversion should be considered
- Magnesium 25–50 mg/kg (to max. of 2 g) IV infusion over several minutes. Indicated in documented hypomagnesemia or torsade de pointes regardless of cause (Advanced Life Support Group 2006)

- Procainamide Loading dose is 15 mg/kg IV given slowly over 30–60 min with ECG and BP monitoring. Stop the infusion if QRS widens or hypotension occurs (Advanced Life Support Group 2006)
- (Lidocaine (lignocaine) 1% 0.1 ml/kg may be considered in VF or VT but is only recommended when amiodarone is unavailable.)

In emergencies it is often difficult to establish intravenous access in infants and children, so consider intraosseous access.

Vagal manoeuvres

These include:

- Application of rubber glove filled with iced water over face – or wrapping infant in towel and immersing face in iced water for 5 seconds
- One-sided carotid sinus massage
- Valsalva manoeuvre, e.g. blowing hard through a straw
- **Do not use ocular pressure in infants or children** as may cause damage.

Sinus tachycardia or supraventricular tachycardia? (Advanced Life Support Group 2006)

- Sinus tachycardia is typically characterised by heart rate of less than 200 bpm in infants and children whereas infants with supraventricular tachycardia (SVT) usually have a heart rate greater than 220 bpm
- P waves may be difficult to identify in both sinus tachycardia and SVT once the ventricular rate exceeds 200 bpm. If P waves are identifiable, they are usually upright in leads I and AVF in sinus tachycardia while they are negative in leads II, III and AVF in SVT
- In sinus tachycardia, the heart rate varies from beat to beat and is often responsive to stimulation, but there is no beat to beat variability in SVT
- Termination of SVT is abrupt whereas the heart rate gradually slows in sinus tachycardia in response to treatment
- A history consistent with shock (e.g. gastroenteritis or septicaemia) is usually present with sinus tachycardia.

USE OF THE DEFIBRILLATOR

The defibrillator can be used both for defibrillation and synchronised cardioversion. All oxygen should be removed from the area before using the defibrillator.

Defibrillation

- is the definitive treatment for ventricular fibrillation (VF) or pulseless ventricular tachycardia (VT) (American Heart Association 1997)

- is the passage of an electrical current through the heart
- is an asynchronous depolarisation of a critical mass of myocardial cells to allow spontaneous reorganised myocardial depolarisation to resume.

When using a manual defibrillator, the shock energy for defibrillation in children is 4 J/kg for all shocks (Resuscitation Council (UK) 2005)

Automated external defibrillators

- A standard automated external defibrillator (AED) can be used for all children over 8 years
- Purpose made pads or programmes that attenuate the energy output of AED are recommended for children between 1 and 8 years
- If no such system or manually adjusted machine is available, an unmodified machine may be used for children over 1 year
- There is insufficient evidence to support a recommendation for or against the use of AEDs in children less than 1 year old.

Resuscitation Council (UK) 2005

Shock sequence

For VF/pulseless VT, one defibrillating shock rather than three 'stacked' shocks is now recommended. This new recommendation for the sequence of defibrillation in children is based on extrapolated data from adult and experimental studies with biphasic devices. Evidence shows a high rate of success for first-shock conversion of ventricular fibrillation (Van Alem et al 2003). Furthermore, interruption of chest compression reduces coronary perfusion pressure, myocardial viability and the chance of successful defibrillation. (Resuscitation Council (UK) 2005).

Synchronised cardioversion

- is the treatment of choice in patients who have tachyarrhythmias, e.g. supraventricular tachycardia, ventricular tachycardia with palpable pulses, atrial fibrillation and atrial flutter, who are seen to be cardio-vascularly compromised (American Heart Association 1997)
- results in depolarisation of the myocardium but provides depolarisation that is timed with the patient's own intrinsic electrical activity.

Initial dose: 1 J/kg
   Subsequent dose will be 2 J/kg (Advanced Life Support Group 2006)
   The discharge buttons on the paddles must be pressed and held for several QRS complexes when cardioverting.

Choice of paddle

- Infant paddles: 4.5 cm, should be used for infants up to 1 year of age or up to 10 kg in weight
- Adult paddles: 8–13 cm, should be used in patients older than 1 year of age and more than 10 kg in weight.

Defibrillation pads

Defibrillation pads are recommended for use rather than electrode gel or KY jelly.

Electrode paddles should be placed so that the heart is in between them. Anterior to posterior electrode and pad position is superior but difficult. Normally, one pad is placed on the upper right chest below the clavicle and the other to the left of the left nipple in the anterior axillary line.

SHOCK

This is defined as inadequate delivery of oxygen and metabolic substrates to meet the metabolic demands of the tissues, which results in inadequate organ and tissue perfusion. This in turn can lead to anaerobic metabolism, lactic acidosis, multisystem organ failure and death.

Usually, shock is associated with low cardiac output but in early septic shock there may be a high-output state with bounding pulses. At this stage there is low systemic vascular resistance and increased blood flow to the skin but there may be a mismatch in distribution of blood flow to the tissues. This can result in tissue hypoxia and eventually a lactic acidosis.

In shock with a low cardiac output there is an increased sympathetic drive, raising the systemic vascular resistance, maintaining the blood pressure and hence perfusion. This diverts blood flow away from non-essential areas, e.g. skin and gut, to increase flow to essential areas, e.g. brain and heart. Clinically a patient in this state will appear pale, feel cool to the touch and have poor peripheral perfusion (American Heart Association 1997).

Shock may be:

- hypovolaemic
- cardiogenic
- septic
- neurogenic
- anaphylactic.

A child in shock will require cardiovascular support with fluid resuscitation and/or inotropic support.

It is useful to classify shock as either compensated or decompensated. See Table 1.2 for classification of haemorrhagic shock.

Compensated shock

(↓ cardiac output, normal blood pressure and ↑ systemic vascular resistance index.)

Table 1.2   Classification of haemorrhagic shock: the effect on five systems

Degree of shock	I: Very mild – haemorrhage, <15% blood volume loss	II: Mild – haemorrhage, 15–25% blood volume loss	III: Moderate – haemorrhage, 26–39% blood volume loss	IV: Severe – haemorrhage, >40% blood volume loss
Cardiovascular	Heart rate normal or mildly raised, normal pulses, normal blood pressure	Tachycardia, peripheral pulses may be diminished, normal blood pressure	Significant tachycardia, thready peripheral pulses, hypotension	Severe tachycardia, thready central pulses, significant hypotension
Respiratory	Normal pH, rate normal	Normal pH, tachypnoea	Metabolic acidosis, moderate tachypnoea	Significant acidosis, severe tachypnoea
Central nervous system	Slightly anxious	Irritable, confused, combative	Irritable or lethargic, diminished pain response	Lethargic, coma
Skin	Warm, pink, capillary refill time brisk (<2 s)	Cool extremities, mottling, delayed capillary refill time (>2 s)	Cool extremities, mottling or pallor, prolonged capillary refill time	Cool extremities, pallor or cyanosis
Kidneys	Normal urine output	Oliguria, increased specific gravity	Oliguria, increased urea	Anuria

Source: modified from American College of Surgeons 1989 and as cited in Hazinski 1992 Fleischer G R, Ludwig S 1988 Textbook of pediatric emergency medicine, 2nd edn. © Lippincott Williams & Wilkins, reproduced with permission.

The child will have a tachycardia and signs of poor peripheral perfusion, e.g. increased capillary refill time, but will have a normal blood pressure at this stage. The child may have a normal level of consciousness but some signs of inadequate tissue perfusion may become apparent, e.g. increasing lactic acidosis.

Decompensated shock

(↓ cardiac output, ↓ blood pressure as ↑ systemic vascular resistance index no longer able to compensate.)

The child will now be hypotensive with weak or absent central pulses and will have an increasing metabolic acidosis, increased capillary refill, a decreased urine output and an altered level of consciousness, reflective of poor end-organ perfusion. This child will need immediate resuscitation as cardiopulmonary arrest will occur if no treatment is given.

Management of shock

- 100% oxygen
- Assess airway and breathing, using adjuncts as necessary
- Establish vascular access – intravenous or intraosseous if necessary
- Use volume expanders and inotropic drugs as required
- Monitor closely.

INTRAOSSEOUS ACCESS

Intraosseous access uses the vascular network in long bones to transport fluids or drugs from the medullary cavity into the circulation.

Sites for intraosseous infusions include the proximal tibia and the medial malleolus.

Advantages of intraosseous access

- Quick, safe and easy to insert
- Medication can be given in the same dose as the intravenous route
- Absorption time has been found to be as effective as intravenous injections in maintaining drug levels.

Contraindications

Not recommended for use:

- on recently fractured bones
- in osteogenesis imperfecta.

Do not give the drug bretylium via the intraosseous route.

Guidelines on insertion of intraosseous needle in proximal tibia

- Immobilise limb and paint with antiseptic
- Use local anaesthetic down to the periosteum if required, i.e. if patient is conscious
- Use landmarks to assess correct placement
- Palpate tibial tuberosity and grasp the medial aspect of the tibia with the thumb – the optimal site of insertion is halfway between these points and 1–2 cm distal (Spivey 1987)
- The needle is inserted perpendicular to the bone at a 15–30° angle towards the foot, i.e. away from the epiphyseal plate

- Apply downward pressure in a boring motion until a 'pop' is heard and resistance suddenly decreases, indicating that the needle has entered the medullary cavity
- The needle should stand up without support
- Penetration from the skin through the cortex is around 1 cm in an infant or child
- Remove inner stylet, and bone marrow content (like blood) should be aspirated to confirm needle placement
- A transparent dressing may be placed around the entry site
- Medication must be administered under pressure and then flushed well.

Complications include needle clotting, extravasation and rarely infection. If fluid is seen to be entering surrounding tissues, stop the infusion immediately, remove needle and apply pressure to the site. An intraosseous needle can remain in place until other intravascular access is obtained.

USEFUL MNEMONICS

Quick assessment tool measuring responsiveness: AVPU
    A   awake
    V   voice
    P   pain
    U   unresponsive
(American Heart Association 1997)

Assessment tool: ABCDEFG
    A   airway
    B   breathing
    C   circulation
    D   don't
    E   ever
    F   forget
    G   glucose – particularly in the fitting child

Common postresuscitation airway complications: DOPE
    D   displacement of endotracheal tube
    O   obstruction of endotracheal tube
    P   pneumothorax
    E   equipment failure

Drugs that can be given via endotracheal tube: LEAN
    L   lidocaine (lignocaine)
    E   epinephrine (adrenaline)
    A   atropine
    N   naloxone

NEWBORN RESUSCITATION

Paediatric intensive care nurses are not often required to resuscitate newborn infants but do need to know the principles if required to do so. Figure 1.6 lists resuscitative procedures in stages: every infant will require the first stage but few will need to proceed to the final stages. Remember: Airway, Breathing, Circulation.

The Apgar score

The Apgar score was developed to indicate a baby's condition at 1 and 5 min after birth. Resuscitation should not be delayed while scores are

Fig 1.6 Algorithm: newborn life support (with permission from Resuscitation Council (UK) 2005)

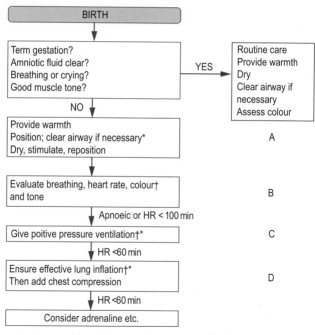

† Consider supplemental oxygen at this stage if cyanosis persists
* Tracheal intubation may be considered at several steps

AT ALL STAGES, ASK.......DO YOU NEED HELP??

Table 1.3	Apgar score				
Score	Heart rate	Respirations	Muscle tone	Response to stimulation	Colour
0	Absent	Absent	Flaccid	None	White/blue
1	Slow <100/min	Gasping/ irregular	Some flexion	Facial grimace	Pink body, blue extremities
2	>100/min	Good/regular	Active movements	Cry/cough	Completely pink

Source: adapted Hull & Johnston 1996.

Age of baby/child	Heart rate (beats/min)	Blood pressure (mmHg)		Respiratory rate (breaths/min)
		Systolic	Diastolic	
Newborn (3 kg)	100–180	50–70	25–45	30–60
Infant	100–160	85–105	55–65	30–60
Toddler	80–110	95–105	55–65	24–40
Preschool	70–110	95–110	55–65	22–34
School age	65–110	95–110	55–70	18–30
Adolescent	60–90	110–130	65–80	12–16

Table 1.4 Normal vital signs – normal values of heart rate, blood pressure and respiratory rate

Source: adapted from Hazinski 1992.

calculated but some knowledge of the scoring system is useful. The maximum score is 10 for a pink, responsive baby who has normal heart rate and respiratory rate, and the minimum score is 0 for a totally unresponsive baby who has no cardiorespiratory function. A score is given to each of five categories as shown in Table 1.3. Table 1.4 shows normal vital signs for infants and children.

MANAGEMENT OF ANAPHYLAXIS

Anaphylaxis is a severe, life-threatening allergic reaction that all nursing and medical staff should know how to treat. A child may present to hospital with an anaphylactic reaction to food products, bee stings, drugs, etc. In hospital, however, anaphylaxis may be caused by latex, blood products, colloids, radiocontrast media or drugs (Ryder & Waldmann 2003). A spectrum of reactions may occur from minor clinical changes to acute cardiovascular collapse and death. A child may present with several of the signs and these may include:

- hypotension
- bradycardia
- tachycardia
- dysrhythmias
- cardiac arrest
- bronchospasm
- laryngeal obstruction
- periorbital oedema
- generalised oedema
- rash
- urticaria
- nausea, vomiting
- diarrhoea
- hoarseness, dry cough
- sneezing
- shortness of breath
- metallic taste in mouth
- chest tightness
- flushing
- feeling faint
- aura of doom (Sampson 2003).

Management includes ABC approach and:

- stop administration of any agent likely to have caused anaphylaxis
- call for help
- maintain airway, give 100% oxygen, intubate and ventilate if necessary
- give adrenaline (epinephrine) via IM route to terminate reaction and repeat after 5 min if required (In one study (Korenblat et al 1999) >35% of patients presenting with varying symptoms of anaphylaxis required more than one dose of adrenaline)
- give intravenous fluids to treat hypotension
- give bronchodilators to reverse bronchospasm
- give antihistamines, e.g. chlorpheniramine IV
- give corticosteroids, e.g. hydrocortisone IV
- consider giving other antihistamine, e.g. ranitidine
- monitor responses, re-evaluate ABC.

Dose of IM adrenaline for acute anaphylaxis

All ages $10\,\mu g/kg$ ($0.01\,ml/kg$ of 1:1000) (Guy's, St Thomas', King's College and University Lewisham Hospitals 2005).

REFERENCES

Advanced Life Support Group 2006 Advanced paediatric life support. The practical approach, 4th edn. BMJ Publishing Group, London

American College of Surgeons 1989 Advanced trauma life support course. American College of Surgeons, Chicago, IL

American Heart Association 1997 Pediatric advanced life support, 3rd edn. American Heart Association, Dallas, TX

Fleisher G R, Ludwig S 1988 Textbook of pediatric emergency medicine, 2nd edn. Williams & Wilkins, Baltimore, MD

Guy's, St Thomas', King's College and University Lewisham Hospitals 2005 Paediatric formulary, 7th edn. Guy's, St Thomas' and Lewisham Hospitals, London

Hazinski M F (ed) 1992 Nursing care of the critically ill child, 2nd edn. Mosby Year Book, St Louis, MO

Hull D, Johnston D I 1996 Essential paediatrics, 3rd edn. Churchill Livingstone, Edinburgh

Korenblat P, Lundie MJ, Dankner RE, Day JH 1999 A retrospective study of epinephrine administration for anaphylaxis: how many doses are needed? Allergy and Asthma Proceedings 20: 383–386

Ryder SA, Waldmann C 2003 Anaphylaxis. Care Crit Ill 19: 174–176

Resuscitation Council (UK) 2005 Resuscitation guidelines 2005. Resuscitation Council (UK), London

Sampson HA 2003 Anaphylaxis and emergency treatment. Pediatrics 111: 1601–1608

Spivey W H 1987 Intraosseous infusions. J Pediatr 111: 639–643

Van Alem AP, Chapman FW, Lank P et al 2003 A prospective, randomised and blinded comparison of first shock success of monophasic and biphasic waveforms in out-of-hospital cardiac arrest. Resuscitation 58, 17–24

FURTHER READING

British Medical Journal 1993 Advanced paediatric life support. British Medical Journal, London

Blumer J L 1990 A practical guide to pediatric intensive care, 3rd edn. C V Mosby, St Louis, MO

Jevon P 2004 Paediatric advanced life support. A practical guide. Butterworth-Heinemann, London

Miccolo M A 1990 Intraosseous infusion. Crit Care Nurse 10(10): 35–47

Versmold H 1981 Aortic blood pressure during the first 12 hours of life in infants with birthweight 610–4220 g. Pediatrics 67–107

Useful website

www.resus.org.uk

AIRWAY, ACID–BASE AND VENTILATION

2

In children it is respiratory failure as opposed to cardiac failure that is often the primary reason for resuscitation. Early recognition and treatment may prevent full cardiopulmonary arrest. Knowledge of the anatomy of the respiratory system in infants and children clarifies the reasons why this occurs. Normal respiratory rates are shown in Box 2.1.

ANATOMY OF THE PAEDIATRIC RESPIRATORY SYSTEM

- Large head, short neck with cartilaginous tracheal rings, which can collapse, causing airway obstruction
- Face and mandible small and underdeveloped in infants
- Relatively large tongue and perhaps loose teeth
- The anterior commissure of the glottis is directed caudally and the infant trachea is angled posteriorly, which may hamper the easy passage of the endotracheal tube
- Larynx is high and anterior (at level of 2nd and 3rd cervical vertebrae in infants compared with 5th and 6th vertebrae in adults)
- Cricoid ring is the narrowest part of the airway as opposed to the larynx in adults
- Compliant rib cage, which can lead to inefficiency in inspiration resulting in increased work of breathing
- Poorly developed intercostal muscles with few type 1 fatigue-resistant fibres, which increases the likelihood of respiratory failure secondary to fatigue
- Protuberant abdomen with caudally displaced diaphragm, which impedes efficient contraction.

Box 2.1   Normal respiratory rates

<1 year: 30–40 breaths/min
2–5 years: 20–30 breaths/min
5–12 years: 15–20 breaths/min
>12 years: 12–16 breaths/min
At rest, tachypnoea indicates that increased ventilation is needed because of either lung or airway disease or metabolic acidosis.

Some infants are obligate nose-breathers. The ability to breathe orally appears to be acquired between 31 and 34 weeks postconception when the baby also acquires the ability to coordinate sucking and swallowing, but Miller et al (1985) found that only 78% of term babies could sustain oral breathing in response to nasal occlusion. They have narrow nasal passages, which are easily obstructed by mucus. Preterm infants have been found to have increased airway resistance and interrupted periods of oral airway obstruction when they breathe orally (Miller et al 1986).

In children aged 3–8 years, adenotonsillar hypertrophy is a common problem, which tends to cause obstruction, and there may be difficulty when the nasal route is used to pass tracheal or gastric tubes.

Oxygenation

This can be assessed by looking at the child's tongue or oral mucosa but can be measured using pulse oximetry or blood gas analysis. In a critically ill child it is important to elicit:

- haemoglobin concentration (Hb)
- oxygen saturation (S_aO_2)
- arterial oxygen content.

Children may be able to cope with mild hypoxia for a short time by increasing their cardiac output but, when they become unable to compensate, cardiorespiratory failure will ensue. The following formulae demonstrate the relationships between haemoglobin, oxygen delivery and cardiac output. Oxygen delivery (DO_2) is the amount of oxygen delivered to the tissues per minute

DO_2 = Arterial oxygen content × cardiac output (CO)

Cardiac output = heart rate × stroke volume

Arterial oxygen content ($mlO_2/100\,ml$) = Hb (g/dl) × 1.34 (mlO_2/gHb) × oxyhaemoglobin saturation + ($0.003 × P_aO_2$)

Haemoglobin that is 100% saturated contains 1.34 ml of bound oxygen.
Normal arterial oxygen content is 18–20 ml of O_2 per 100 ml blood.

VENTILATION AND DEFINITION OF TERMS

- **Ventilation** is the process of movement of gas between the lungs and the ambient air
- **Tidal volume** is the volume of gas that is inspired and expired in one normal breath (6 ml/kg)
- **Minute volume** is the quantity of gas expired by the lungs in one minute: minute volume = tidal volume × frequency
- **Functional residual capacity** is the amount of gas that remains in the lungs after normal expiration

- The anatomical dead space (around 30% of each tidal volume) fills the conducting airways and no gas exchange takes place there.

Pulse oximetry

This is a non-invasive, reliable and easy-to-use method of calculating a patient's oxygen saturation. The pulse oximeter consists of a photodetector that is wrapped around a pulsatile tissue bed, i.e. on a finger or toe, or on the ear, and two light-emitting diodes that transmit red and infrared light. Oxygenated and deoxygenated haemoglobin absorb these two lights differently and the haemoglobin saturation (percentage of total haemoglobin oxygenated) is inversely related to the amount of red light absorbed.

The pulse oximeter is thought to be accurate to ±4% when oxygen saturation is 80% or above but below this figure it tends to over-read and may not detect acute changes and severe hypoxaemia. Inaccurate readings may also occur as a result of poor peripheral perfusion, oedema, hypothermia or jaundice, or with abnormal haemoglobins, e.g. methaemoglobin or carboxyhaemoglobin. A raised bilirubin will cause under-reading of the oxygen saturation as the bilirubin absorbs the light but the presence of carboxyhaemoglobin will lead to an overestimation of saturation of the total haemoglobin of blood. The pulse oximeter is also sensitive to movement and this may interfere with readings (Taylor & Whitwam 1986).

Oxyhaemoglobin dissociation curve

The oxyhaemoglobin dissociation curve (Fig. 2.1) shows the non-linear relationship between haemoglobin saturation and the partial pressure of oxygen (P_aO_2). Each molecule of haemoglobin is made up of a protein (globin) and a combination of ferrous iron and protophyrin (haem), of which

Fig 2.1 Oxyhaemoglobin dissociation curve, showing the relationship between haemoglobin saturation and pH

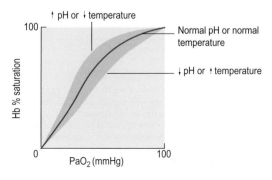

there are four. Each haem group has a different affinity to oxygen. Looking at the oxyhaemoglobin dissociation curve, the first haem group binds moderately easily with oxygen and there is a gentle curve. The second and third haems have the greatest affinity for oxygen and there is a steep slope as the haemoglobin saturation rises with a relatively small change in the P_aO_2. The fourth haem has the greatest difficulty binding to oxygen and so the curve flattens out, relatively less oxygen being taken up per unit change in P_aO_2 as the haemoglobin is reaching near-total saturation, i.e. 97–100%. This occurs when P_aO_2 reaches around 13.3 kPa; there is therefore no additional benefit in keeping a patient's P_aO_2 any higher than this.

If the curve is shifted to the right, then haemoglobin binds less oxygen and is less well saturated at any partial pressure of oxygen. Factors that shift the curve to the right include acidosis, hypercapnia and hyperthermia.

If the curve is shifted to the left, haemoglobin binds more oxygen at any partial pressure of oxygen. Factors that shift the curve to the left include alkalosis, hypocapnia and hypothermia.

Signs of respiratory distress and inadequate ventilation in children

Tachypnoea, cricoid tug, sternal, intercostal or subcostal recession, shoulder rolling, nasal flaring, weak cry, stridor or wheeze, head bobbing, lethargy, decreased responsiveness, irritability, decreased level of consciousness, hypoxaemia, hypercarbia

Late signs: bradycardia, decreased air movement, apnoea or gasping, poor systemic perfusion

UPPER RESPIRATORY TRACT

Common conditions that affect the upper respiratory tract include croup, epiglottitis, tracheal stenosis or malacia and any respiratory condition that leads to an increase in respiratory secretions.

The airway of infants and children is much smaller than that of adults. Poiseuille's law states:

$$resistance \propto 1/radius^4,$$

that is, the resistance to airflow is inversely proportional to the fourth power of the radius. In other words, a small amount of mucus in the airway, oedema or tracheal stenosis will significantly increase resistance to airflow and will increase the work of breathing.

A child with upper airway obstruction will be most comfortable sitting up and leaning forwards, may be anxious, restless, cyanosed, tachypnoeic, have an inspiratory stridor, drool, have nasal flaring and be using the accessory muscles to breathe.

LOWER RESPIRATORY TRACT

Common conditions that affect the lower respiratory tract include bronchiolitis, asthma, pneumonia, foreign body aspiration and respiratory distress syndrome. Bronchospasm, increased mucus production, oedema and inflammation of airway mucosa can lead to diffuse air trapping, decreased air movement, decreased compliance and increased work of breathing. A child with lower respiratory tract disease may have an expiratory wheeze, prolonged expiratory time, be tachypnoeic, cyanotic, use accessory muscles, cough and may have hyperinflated lungs.

ACID–BASE BALANCE AND INTERPRETATION OF BLOOD GASES

pH is a term used to describe the acidity or alkalinity of a solution. The pH scale is based on the concentration of hydrogen ions, expressed in moles per litre, which is the negative logarithm of the hydrogen concentration.

- pH below 7 = an acid solution, which dissociates into H^+ ions (cations) and OH^- ions (anions) with more H^+ ions than OH^- ions
- pH above 7 = an alkaline solution, which dissociates into OH^- ions and H^+ ions with more OH^- ions than H^+ ions.

Three major mechanisms homeostatically control blood pH:

- buffers
- respiration
- renal excretion.

Normal blood pH = 7.35–7.45.
    pH levels of below 6.8 and above 7.8 are typically incompatible with life. See Table 2.1 for normal arterial blood gas values in infants and children.

Buffers

The most important buffer is the carbonic-acid–bicarbonate buffer system in which carbonic acid (H_2CO_3) is the weak acid and sodium bicarbonate ($NaHCO_3$) is the weak base. In solution dissociation occurs:

H_2CO_3	$\rightleftharpoons$	H^+	+	HCO_3^-
Carbonic acid		hydrogen		bicarbonate
$NaHCO_3$	$\rightleftharpoons$	Na^+	+	HCO_3^-
Sodium bicarbonate		sodium		bicarbonate.

If the blood becomes very acidic, the sodium bicarbonate disassociates to buffer the acid, thus increasing concentration of carbonic acid and decreasing sodium bicarbonate, but the net result is an increase in pH (as carbonic acid is weak). If there is a strong base in the blood, i.e. the blood is alkaline, the concentration of sodium bicarbonate increases and carbonic acid is used up as the buffer. Other buffer systems include phosphate, haemoglobin–oxyhaemoglobin and protein buffer systems.

Table 2.1	Normal arterial blood gas values for neonates and children	
	Normal infant/child values	**Normal neonatal values**
pH	7.35–7.45	7.3–7.4
P_{CO_2} (kPa)	4.5–6.0 (35–45 mmHg)	4.6–6.0 (35–45 mmHg)
P_{O_2} (kPa)	10–13 (75–100 mmHg)	7.3–12 (55–90 mmHg)
Bicarbonate (mmol/l)	22–26	18–25
Base (mmol/l)	−2 to +2	−4 to +4

The phosphate buffer system works in a similar way to the carbonic acid system in the red blood cells and the kidney tubular fluids. The haemo-globin–oxyhaemoglobin buffer system buffers carbonic acid in the blood, while the protein buffer system works in the body cells and plasma.

Respiration

Respirations regulate the level of carbon dioxide (CO_2) in body fluids:

$$CO_2 + H_2O \rightleftharpoons H_2CO_3 \rightleftharpoons H^+ + HCO_3^-.$$

The level of P_{CO_2} in the blood gas will signify whether there is a respira-tory component. If the P_{CO_2} is high, this signifies a respiratory acidosis and if it is low, this signifies a respiratory alkalosis. An increased respiratory rate eliminates CO_2 and less H_2CO_3 and H^+ are formed, increasing pH.

Renal secretion

Kidney tubular secretion helps control the pH of blood. If the pH of blood is acidic, there is increased secretion of H^+, which displaces another cation, usually Na^+, which then diffuses from the urine into the tubule cell where it combines with bicarbonate to form sodium bicarbonate, which then gets absorbed into the blood stream. Thus H^+ is lost from the body and the pH becomes less acidic (Tortora & Anagnostakos 1984).

Interpretation of blood gas analyses

The primary problem in an acid–base disorder is defined by its initiat-ing process, which may be metabolic (changes in HCO_3) or respiratory (changes in P_aCO_2). A compensatory response describes the secondary physiological response to the primary disturbance. Box 2.2 lists com-mon causes of acidosis and alkalosis.

To interpret blood gas values (Resuscitation Council (UK) 2004):

- Assess oxygenation – is the child hypoxic?
- Assess pH
  - pH > 7.45 is alkalosis
  - pH < 7.35 is acidosis

Box 2.2 Common causes of acidosis and alkalosis

Respiratory acidosis

Any cause of hypoventilation:

- Obstructive airways disease, e.g. asthma
- CNS depression, e.g. head injury, encephalitis
- Neuromuscular disease, e.g. myasthenia gravis, Guillain–Barré syndrome
- Artificial ventilation

Respiratory alkalosis

Any cause of hyperventilation:

- Psychogenic, e.g. hysteria, pain
- Central, e.g. raised intracranial pressure, meningitis
- Pulmonary, e.g. hypoxia, pulmonary embolus or oedema, pneumonia
- Metabolic, e.g. fever, acute liver failure
- Drugs, e.g. acute salicylate poisoning
- Artificial ventilation

Metabolic acidosis

Normal anion gap:

- Intestinal losses, e.g. diarrhoea
- Renal losses, e.g. renal tubular acidosis

Increased anion gap:

- Overproduction of organic acid, e.g. diabetic ketoacidosis, lactic acidosis
- Decreased ability to conserve HCO_3, e.g. chronic renal failure
- Advanced salicylate, methanol or ethylene glycol poisoning
- Inborn errors of metabolism, e.g. maple syrup urine disease

Metabolic alkalosis

- Excess acid loss, e.g. persistent vomiting as in pyloric stenosis
- Diuretic therapy
- Excess intake of alkali

- Assess respiratory component
  - $P_aCO_2 > 6\,kPa$: respiratory acidosis (or renal compensation for a respiratory alkalosis)
  - $P_aCO_2 < 4.7\,kPa$: respiratory alkalosis (or respiratory compensation for a metabolic acidosis)
- Assess metabolic component
  - $HCO_3 < 22\,mmol/l$: metabolic acidosis (or renal compensation for a respiratory alkalosis)
  - $HCO_3 > 26\,mmol/l$: metabolic alkalosis (or renal compensation for a respiratory acidosis)
- Determine primary disturbance and whether there is any metabolic or respiratory compensation

Table 2.2 Changes in pH, P_aCO_2 and HCO_3 in acid base disorders

Acid–base disorder	pH	P_aCO_2	HCO_3
Respiratory acidosis	↓	↑	N
Metabolic acidosis	↓	N	↓
Respiratory alkalosis	↑	↓	N
Metabolic alkalosis	↑	N	↑
Respiratory acidosis with renal compensation	↓ *	↑	↑
Metabolic acidosis with respiratory compensation	↓ *	↓	↓
Respiratory alkalosis with renal compensation	↑ *	↓	↓
Metabolic alkalosis with respiratory compensation	↑ *	↑	↑
Mixed metabolic and respiratory acidosis	↓	↑	↓
Mixed metabolic and respiratory alkalosis	↑	↓	↑

* If compensation is virtually complete, the pH may be in the normal range – overcompensation does not occur.

Source: Resuscitation Council (UK) 2004.

Metabolic disturbances are compensated acutely by changes in ventilation and chronically by appropriate renal responses. Respiratory disturbances are compensated by renal tubular secretion of hydrogen.

In chronic conditions where PCO_2 is increased, there is renal compensation and retention of bicarbonate, with pH returning to near normal levels. Table 2.2 shows effects of acid base disorders on pH, P_aCO_2 and HCO_3.

Anion gap

It may be useful to calculate the anion gap if the cause of a metabolic acidosis is not known. The anion gap is calculated as the difference between the sum of plasma sodium and potassium and the sum of plasma bicarbonate and chloride concentration:

Anion gap = (sodium + potassium) − (total bicarbonate + chloride).

The normal anion gap ranges from 5–12 mmol/l. A patient who has a metabolic acidosis with a normal anion gap will have lost base, e.g. with diarrhoea. A patient with a metabolic acidosis who has an increased anion gap will have gained acid, e.g. in ketoacidosis (Hinds & Watson 1996). NB. The anion gap will be underestimated with hypoalbuminaemia.

SYSTEMATIC REVIEW OF CHEST X-RAY

This should include:

- Bones and soft tissues
- Mediastinum, including thymus
- Heart and great vessels

Fig 2.2   Chest X-ray interpretation (based on Corne et al 2002)

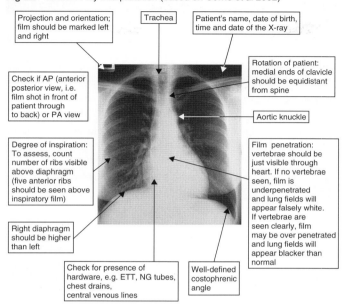

Projection and orientation; film should be marked left and right

Trachea

Patient's name, date of birth, time and date of the X-ray

Check if AP (anterior posterior view, i.e. film shot in front of patient through to back) or PA view

Rotation of patient: medial ends of clavicle should be equidistant from spine

Aortic knuckle

Degree of inspiration: To assess, count number of ribs visible above diaphragm (five anterior ribs should be seen above inspiratory film)

Film penetration: vertebrae should be just visible through heart. If no vertebrae seen, film is underpenetrated and lung fields will appear falsely white. If vertebrae are seen clearly, film may be over penetrated and lung fields will appear blacker than normal

Right diaphragm should be higher than left

Check for presence of hardware, e.g. ETT, NG tubes, chest drains, central venous lines

Well-defined costophrenic angle

- Lungs
- Abdomen.

See Fig. 2.2 chest X-ray interpretation and Figs 2.4–2.8 for striking abnormalities on chest X-ray.

Bones and soft tissue

Observe clavicles, ribs, scapulae and vertebra – follow the edges of each bone to look for fractures or areas of calcification. Look for any enlargement of areas of soft tissue or vertebral abnormalities. Observe if there is any rib crowding which could indicate atelectasis.

Mediastinum including thymus

The thymus is usually apparent on the chest X-ray until the age of around 2 years although it may still be seen in older children up to 4 years (Schelvan et al 2002). It can typically be seen on both sides of the superior mediastinum, has a smooth lateral border and blends inferiorly with the cardiac contour (although sometimes there is a little notch at the junction). The edge of the mediastinum should be clear and a fuzzy edge may suggest consolidation or collapse in the adjacent lung field.

Thymus is absent in DiGeorge's syndrome.

The trachea should be central but deviates slightly to the right around the aortic knuckle. Check the position of the right and left main bronchi (splaying of the left bronchi could indicate left atrial enlargement).

Heart and great vessels

Assess the heart size. This should be around 50% of the cardiothoracic ratio but this is slightly increased in neonates. The heart is usually situated one-third on the right of the spine and two-thirds on the left.

 The thymic shadow may give a false impression of cardiomegaly in infants.

The right heart border on the X-ray is the right atrium of the heart. The left heart border comprises the aorta, the pulmonary arteries, the left atrium and the right ventricle.

(An enlarged right ventricle in the heart may be observed on X-ray if the apex is uplifted. An enlarged left ventricle moves the apex left laterally towards the chest wall.)

Observe and note:

- Heart position and orientation
- Aortic arch orientation
- Size of heart
- Any enlarged chambers or vessels
- Perfusion of lung fields
- Congestion of lung fields
- Other findings, e.g. prosthesis – valves, stents, calcification.

Signs of heart failure on chest X-ray

- Cardiomegaly
- Upper lobe venous equilibration
- Alveolar oedema – 'fluffy appearance'
- Hepatomegaly
- Fluid in fissures and pleural effusions sometimes present.

 Cardiomegaly may not just indicate cardiac failure. You may also need to consider cardiomyopathy and Ebstein's anomaly.

Fig. 2.3 Diagram showing lung lobes and fissures

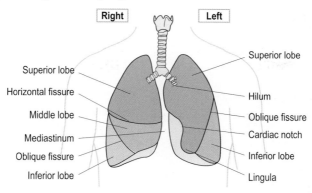

Lungs

Lung fields should appear black in colour, which indicates the presence of air except for the pulmonary vessel markings. The lung fields should be of equal translucency. See Fig. 2.3 showing lung anatomy.

- Identify the horizontal fissures
- Check lung volumes – if asymmetrical consider inhalation of a foreign body, or if hyperinflated, consider bronchiolitis in a baby or asthma in an older child
- Observe for any focal pathology, e.g. mediastinal mass, consolidation or collapse
- Observe for any diffuse abnormality, e.g. pulmonary oedema or fibrosis
- Observe for pulmonary shadows within lung tissue – look for symmetry, i.e. reticular nodular appearance (interstitial fluid), look for reduced pulmonary markings that could indicate bullae (ring-like appearance)
- Observe for extrapulmonary shadows, i.e. outside lung tissue, e.g. pleural effusion, pneumothorax, empyema (loculated white areas).

The right diaphragm should be higher than the left diaphragm (less than 3 cm). The costophrenic angles should be acute, well defined angles and if the cardiophrenic angles (adjacent heart border) are fuzzy and indistinct consider that the adjacent area of lung has collapse/consolidation.

Abdomen

- Check the position of all visible abdominal organs on the X-ray, e.g. for situs solitus
- Check for the gastric air bubble
- Look for air under the diaphragm or obviously dilated loops of bowel.

Striking abnormalities on chest X-ray – what to look out for

Consolidation

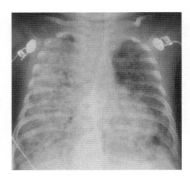

Fig 2.4   This is a term used to describe lung tissue where air filled spaces are replaced by products of disease, e.g. water, pus, mucus or blood.

Radiological findings: shadowing with ill-defined markings, air bronchograms, silhouette sign (where the border of a structure is lost by consolidation), no volume loss.

Atelectasis

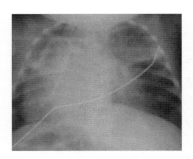

Fig 2.5   This refers to a loss of aeration in the lung, which leads to collapse. It is not usually an infective process but may be caused by a foreign body, aspiration, tumour or mucus plug.

Radiological findings: crowding of ribs, shift of mediastinum usually towards the white lung field, elevation of the hemidiaphragm, compensatory hyperinflation.

Pleural effusion

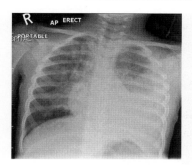

Fig 2.6   This refers to fluid in the pleural space.

Radiological findings: will be different in erect and supine films; the effusion will be white in colour and a visible meniscus may be present. Look for air bronchograms as this finding may lead you to suspect consolidation rather than effusion. An absence of mediastinal shift suggests an effusion but collapse with an effusion can occur with some mediastinal shift.

Pneumothorax

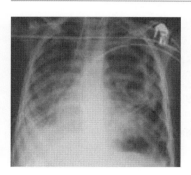

Fig 2.7   This refers to air within the pleural space.

Radiological findings: black area with loss of vascular markings to the pleural edge.

Tension pneumothorax

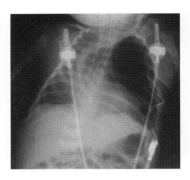

Fig 2.8   If air enters the pleural space during inspiration and cannot leave during expiration, this will lead to a rapid increase in pressure and a life-threatening tension pneumothorax.

Radiological findings: a hyperlucent (black) lung field with a complete absence of vascular markings on that side, shift of mediastinum to the opposite side and flattening of the ipsilateral diaphragm.

Life-threatening tension pneumothorax requires immediate intervention – placing a large-bore cannula in the second intercostal space in the mid-clavicular line on the side of the pneumothorax then following this up with a pleural drain. It does not need an X-ray urgently, it requires intervention first.

Lung perfusion

An X-ray must be normally penetrated to be able to see if lungs are under- or overperfused. In a normally penetrated X-ray, vertebrae should bevisible through the cardiac silhouette but not through the liver. Under-perfused lung fields are blacker to the edge (oligaemic). Overperfused lung fields have increased vessel markings to the peripheries (hyperaemic).

MEANS AND METHODS OF OXYGEN DELIVERY

This can be divided into high- or low-flow methods.

Low flow

Mask, e.g. Venturi can give wide range of concentrations, from 35–60% oxygen with a flow rate of 6–10 l/min. The inspired oxygen can only reach 60% as air mixes with oxygen through the exhalation ports in the side of the mask. A minimum flow of 6 l/min must be used to maintain an increased oxygen concentration to prevent rebreathing of exhaled carbon dioxide.

Nasal cannula: A maximum flow rate of 2 l/min is usually prescribed, as higher flow rates will irritate the nasopharynx. However this could vary up to 4 l/min according to manufacturers' instructions.

Table 2.3	Oxygen concentration versus flow rates
Oxygen concentration (%)	**Oxygen flow (litres)**
28	4–5
31	6
35	8
40	9
60	10

High flow

Headbox: Able to achieve an inspired oxygen concentration of 80–90%. Always use an oxygen analyser and titrate oxygen concentration to patient requirement. The flow rate must be 10–15 l/min to prevent accumulation of carbon dioxide (Table 2.3).

Oxygenation index

The oxygenation index (OI) is a tool used to assess the degree of hypoxia related to the amount of mechanical support and the inspired oxygen tension. It can be calculated:

$$OI = \frac{\text{Mean airways pressure} \times (\text{fraction of inspired oxygen} \times 100)}{PaO_2 \times 7.5 \, mmHg}$$

It is sometimes calculated when patients are nearing maximal conventional ventilator settings and clinicians are considering adjunct therapy, e.g. high-frequency oscillation (HFOV) or extracorporeal membrane oxygenation (ECMO). It is useful to observe trends in OI and response to interventions.

In the adult population with adult respiratory distress syndrome (ARDS), HFOV should be considered when OI is 22–46, but OI above this figure in patients who were not on HFOV led to 100% mortality (Fort et al 1997). ECMO may be considered in the neonatal population when OI is $\geqslant 40$.

INDICATIONS FOR ASSISTED VENTILATION

Apnoea, respiratory distress with either increasing PCO_2 or decreasing pH and poor oxygenation.

MODES OF VENTILATION

Non-invasive ventilation

There are several options for non-invasive ventilation (NIV). These include:

- Nasal CPAP, e.g. Infant flow™ driver

- Biphasic cuirass ventilation (BCV)
- Biphasic positive airways pressure (BiPaP™).

Non-invasive ventilation summary of recommendations (British Thoracic Society Standards of Care Committee 2002)

- NIV has been shown to be an effective treatment for acute hypercapnic respiratory failure. Facilities should be available 24 h/d in hospitals likely to admit such patients.
- NIV should not be used as a substitute for tracheal intubation and invasive ventilation when this would be more appropriate.
- Benefits of NIV have been demonstrated mainly in patients with a respiratory acidosis (pH < 7.35). ABG should be measured in most breathless patients.
- ABG tensions improve rapidly in many patients receiving maximum medical treatment and appropriate supplementary oxygen. Therefore a repeat sample should be taken after a short interval to see if NIV is still indicated.
- There should be a low threshold for measuring ABG tensions in patients with neuromuscular diseases, chest wall deformity, obesity or acute confusional states who may be in respiratory failure without significant breathlessness.

Infant Flow™ Driver

Infant Flow™ Driver provides nasal CPAP via nasal prongs or a mask. This is designed to reduce the work of breathing by providing active assistance on both inspiratory and expiratory phases of the respiratory cycle. (This differs from PEEP, which provides positive end expiratory pressure only.) CPAP restores functional residual capacity and allows normal breathing with normal pressures.

Follow manufacturer's instructions before use:

Five core principles –

- Ensure there is a good seal
- Ensure the equipment remains in a good, stable position
- Ensure the baby remains comfortable
- Monitor the baby and document observations
- Ensure a holistic approach is used.

See Fig. 2.9.

Step-by-step leak test –

- Assemble and attach circuit to driver
- Adjust flow to 8 l/min
- Occlude prongs or mask
- Ensure pressure is 4–5 cmH$_2$O.

It is advisable to use an orogastric tube instead of a nasogastric tube if one is required as nasogastric tubes impede fixation and significantly add to the work of breathing.

Fig 2.9 Step by step fixation technique (with permission from VIASYS Healthcare Clinical Training Book: The Infant Flow System)

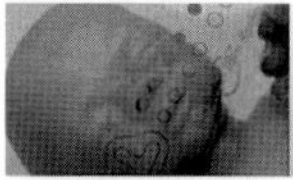	**Step 1** Select correct size of patient interface – nasal prong or nasal mask	Use nose guide provided to select the correct size of prong or mask. The shaded area indicates the infant's nares size. The clear area indicates the size of the prong/mask. Insert prong/mask into the generator.
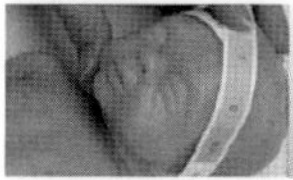	**Step 2** Select bonnet	Use tape to measure for appropriate bonnet size. Measure from center of forehead to nape of the neck and back to forehead. Use bonnet size guide to select appropriate size.
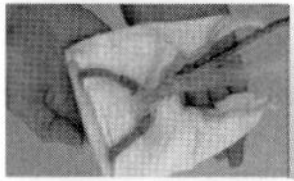	**Step 3** Fixation technique – generator to bonnet	Loosely weave the generator straps through the buttonholes starting inside the bonnet with the lowest color-coded buttonhole. Place generator on top of the bonnet above the central Velcro tie.
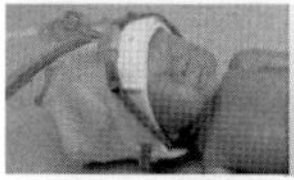	**Step 4** Fixation technique – bonnet placement	Support generator on bonnet. Gently place the bonnet on infant's head, checking ears are in a normal position. Pull the bonnet well down over the infant's head. The button holes will be positioned over the infant's ears.
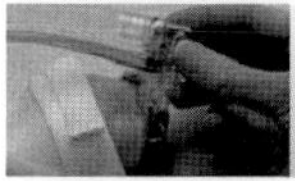	**Step 5** Fixation technique – generator placement	Lift the generator from the top of bonnet and bring towards the infant's nose. Gently insert the prongs or mask into position to deliver NCPAP. Take the generator straps horizontally across the infant's cheeks and secure, but **do not over tighten**.
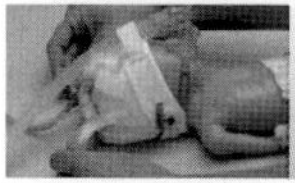	**Step 6** Fixation technique – adjust and secure	Support the generator while securing all three tubings using the central Velcro tie. Split the inspiratory and pressure lines and secure with secondary Velcro ties. Tie off open end of bonnet.
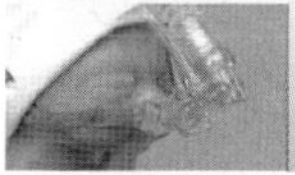	**Step 7** Final check	Check: Prongs/mask in position, no pressure or squashing of nose; • eyes are clearly visible, ears in normal position • generator is stable and secure • infant is receiving required level of nCPAP

Biphasic cuirass ventilation

Biphasic cuirass ventilation − RTX Respirator (described below) and Hayek Oscillator − is a non-invasive form of ventilation that actively controls both the inspiratory and expiratory phases of the respiratory cycle. Increasing pressure within the cuirass causes chest compression, which leads to expiration, while decreasing pressures within the cuirass leads to chest expansion and inspiration. BCV helps to maintain and redevelop respiratory muscles and improves cardiac output.

Suggested clinical uses include:

- Acute respiratory failure
- Chronic obstructive pulmonary disease
- Decompensated obstructive sleep apnoea
- Ventilatory failure due to neuromuscular disorders.

The RTX Respirator has seven modes of operation:

- **Monitor mode** used to monitor patient's breathing pattern, ECG and pulse oximeter − but respirator on standby, i.e. gives no support
- **Continuous negative mode** increases lung volume by creating continuous negative chamber pressure while the patient is spontaneously breathing
- **Control mode** controls both inspiratory and expiratory phases of breathing through changes to frequency, I/E ratio, inspiratory and expiratory pressure
- **Respiratory trigger mode** initiated by the patient's inspiration. The trigger can be set to airway or the cuirass and there is a minimum back up rate.
- **Respiratory synchronised mode** allows patients to breath at their own rate but their inspiratory and expiratory efforts are triggers for the respirator and thus full synchronisation with their respirations is achieved. A minimum back up rate can be set.
- **ECG-triggered mode** the respiratory cycle is synchronised to the cardiac cycle − exhalation to systole and inhalation to diastole (NB. This ECG is a rhythm strip only with no arrhythmia detection alarms)
- **Secretion clearance mode** can be set in vibration mode to loosen secretions or cough mode, which creates a cough-like effect.

Technical capability:
- Frequency range: 6–1200 cycles/min
- I/E ratio: 1:6–6:1
- Maximum inspiratory pressure: $-50\,cmH_2O$
- Maximum expiratory pressure: $+50\,cmH_2O$.

Plastic cuirass: There are seven different sizes of paediatric cuirass and four adult sizes. The cuirass should fit from the axillae to at least below the umbilicus. The cuirass must create an airtight seal around the chest.

Select the largest cuirass that can be closed over the patient without leakage. Ideally the patient should wear a loose fitting garment. See Fig. 2.10 for application of cuirass.

Fig 2.10 Application of cuirass (with permission from Medivent Ltd 2002)

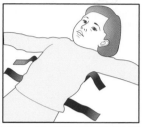

Place the straps under the patient.

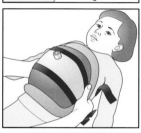

Pull the sides of the cuirass open and place over patient's chest and abdomen.

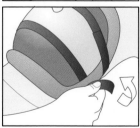

Attach the straps under the patient to the cuirass and ensure that there is an airtight seal by running finger between foam and patient.

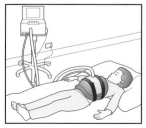

Attach cuirass to respirator. Patient can be cared for lying in bed or in a seated position.

Biphasic positive airways pressure

Biphasic positive airways pressure (BiPaP™, Medic Aid Ltd) is non-invasive, intermittent, positive-pressure-assisted ventilation that can either be triggered by the patient or fully controlled via a mask or tracheostomy. It is pressure-support ventilation with positive end expiratory pressure (PEEP).

BiPaP™ can give two levels of respiratory support, continuous positive airways pressure (CPAP), sometimes known as expiratory positive airways pressure (EPAP), and inspiratory positive airways pressure (IPAP).

CPAP:
- helps keep airways open
- improves alveolar gas exchange
- improves oxygenation
- increases lung volume.

IPAP:
- supports inspiratory effort and decreases work of breathing
- improves tidal volumes
- improves CO_2 removal.

Indications:
- Reduced respiratory effort
- Upper airways obstruction
- Airway recruitment tool.

Absolute contraindications:
- Uncooperative patient
- Recent facial, oesophageal or gastric surgery
- Craniofacial trauma or burns
- Fixed anatomical abnormality of nasopharynx.

Caution in patients with respiratory arrest or with cardiorespiratory instability. Consider if NIV is the best option.

Precautions:
- Nasogastric tube in situ – particularly if using a full face mask
- Use Granuflex/Duoderm/protective layer over vulnerable areas, e.g. bridge of nose, ears.

Most circuits are disposable. Circuits will contain:

- a pressure line, which may or may not be employed depending on the machine in use
- an expiratory port built in near patient end, which must not be occluded

- a filter attached to the outflow port of the machine
- an appropriate-sized mask
- oxygen port, which attaches to a flow meter if required.

Selecting the appropriate mask is vital to the success of BiPaP™. Use either nasal mask or full face mask.

- **Nasal mask** Use the size gauge to measure for the correct mask. Aim for the smallest fitting mask without sacrificing length from the bridge of the nose. Nasal masks can be used as full face masks on small children
- **Full face masks** This should fit from the bridge of the nose to just below the bottom lip. Use the foam spacer to attach to the top of the mask to bridge the gap from the forehead to the upright strut of the mask.

Starting BiPaP™: The spontaneous mode is the most common mode but a back-up rate can be used if the patient has apnoeas. NB. If IPAP and EPAP are set at the same level, the patient receives CPAP.

Give a full explanation to the child and family. Switch on the machine before applying the mask. Hold the mask on the child's face to allow the child to get used to it before strapping it on. Then apply and tighten the straps firmly to eliminate large leaks. Tighten top straps then bottom straps together. Slowly increase pressures to a comfortable, therapeutic level or as the child's condition determines.

Stop BiPaP™ if:
- worsening encephalopathy or agitation
- inability to clear secretions
- haemodynamic instability
- worsening oxygenation
- progressive hypercapnia

as patient will need further assessment and possible intubation and ventilation, **or**
- if the child's condition has improved, then intolerance of BiPaP™ may indicate that it is no longer required.

Invasive ventilatory modes via tracheal intubation

There are many modes of ventilation that can be used on a child requiring ventilatory assistance. One classification distinguishes those with an intact respiratory drive who require minimal help, e.g. pressure support mode or even just continuous positive airways pressure, from others who require more controlled ventilatory support, e.g. in a mandatory ventilation mode. Various modes are explained, highlighting some of the advantages and disadvantages. (Information from 'Pressure-control ventilation' to 'Positive end expiratory pressure (PEEP)' is adapted from Siemens Medical Engineering 1993, with permission.)

Pressure-control ventilation

- Used in neonates and infants with poor lung compliance and increased airway resistance
- Flow and pressure are controlled by ventilator settings
- Time cycled: each respiratory cycle is made up by setting the inspired and expired time in seconds
- Continuous flow of gas allowing the infant to interbreathe between ventilator breaths
- Time-triggered ventilator breaths, which may be synchronised or mandatory breaths depending on the ventilator setting
- Volumes are not measured but are dependent on chest compliance and resistance.

The advantage of pressure-controlled ventilation is the avoidance of high airway pressures, but the disadvantage is that there is no guarantee of volume delivered.

Volume-control ventilation

- Used mainly in children over 10 kg
- Tidal volume between 10 and 15 ml/kg
- Preset tidal volume, inspired minute volume, frequency of breaths and inspiratory time
- Pressure is not set but dependent on lung compliance and resistance
- Can be used in many modes.

Controlled mandatory ventilation (CMV)

- Patient receives a preset number of ventilator-generated breaths at a preset tidal volume, at mandatory intervals
- Gas flow is present so that the patient may breathe spontaneously in between each mandatory breath.

Synchronised intermittent mandatory ventilation (SIMV)

- Provides preset breaths at a preset tidal volume, but the breaths are synchronised with the patient's initiation of inspiration. The patient may take additional breaths.

Pressure support (PS)

- Patient initiates a breath, thus generating negative pressure, and then the ventilator provides a breath with preset airways pressure; the amount of negative pressure required to generate a breath is set by altering the trigger sensitivity
- There is no back-up rate
- Patient must generate own rate, inspiratory time and tidal volume.

(Using the Servo ventilators, the trigger is measured in cmH_2O. Thus a trigger of 2 cmH_2O below positive end expiratory pressure (PEEP) requires minimal effort before a breath is delivered but -5 requires more effort. Using the SLE ventilator, the trigger is measured in minimum and maximum sensitivity; therefore, if the trigger is set at 5, this is the most sensitive setting, requiring the least effort to trigger a breath.)

Patient trigger ventilation (PTV)

- Back-up rate is set on the CMV setting using preset inspiratory time, peak inspiratory pressure (PIP) and PEEP to act as a safety mechanism in case of apnoea
- Patient initiates a breath, generates negative pressure and the ventilator will deliver the preset breath at a rate determined by the patient
- Trigger sensitivity must be set to determine the amount of negative pressure required in order that a breath be delivered.

SIMV pressure control and pressure support (SIMV PC & PS)

- Combination of controlled and support ventilation
- Synchronised mandatory breaths at preset rate/min with controlled pressures
- When patient interbreathes and generates a negative pressure, these triggered breaths are pressure-supported (this avoids high airway pressures but the volumes cannot be set).

SIMV volume control and pressure support (SIMV VC & PS)

- Ventilator delivers synchronised mandatory volume-controlled breaths
- When patient makes respiratory effort in between these breaths and generates a negative pressure, these will be pressure supported, i.e. breath is delivered to the preset pressure support set above PEEP.

Pressure-regulated volume control (PRVC)

- Combines the advantages of both pressure and volume control
- Set the tidal and minute volume plus the upper pressure limit
- This mode delivers volumes set with lower inspiratory pressures than in volume control mode.

Volume support (VS)

- Set tidal volumes
- In case of apnoea, preset rate, tidal and minute volumes are set in PRVC and will be delivered and the ventilator will alarm
- Gives lowest inspiratory pressure support to deliver the preset tidal volume

- If lung compliance changes, inspiratory support pressure will be regulated to deliver set tidal volumes.

Automode ventilation (Servo 300A)

Pressure or volume support ventilation with a back up rate if the patient is apnoeic. Automode is suitable for patients with respiratory drive who can trigger the ventilator but who require back up. Ventilation remains in support mode as long as the patient breathes spontaneously. If apnoea occurs, ventilation automatically takes over in control mode giving pre-set back up breaths until the patient makes a respiratory effort, when it switches back to support mode.

Continuous positive airways pressure (CPAP)

- Used in patients with intact respiratory drive, as no back-up rate
- Increases or maintains lung volume, opens atelectatic areas of the lungs and can increase functional residual capacity (FRC)
- Patient generates respiratory rate, inspiratory time, tidal volume and peak inspiratory pressure but CPAP maintains a positive end expiratory pressure at all times.

Positive end expiratory pressure (PEEP)

- Increases FRC and maintains lung recruitment
- Improves alveolar ventilation
- Increases arterial oxygen content
- Increases intrathoracic pressure and may impede systemic venous return and thus cardiac output
- High PEEP, i.e. above 8, may impede cerebral venous return, which may increase intercranial pressure.

HIGH-FREQUENCY VENTILATION

This is defined by high-frequency, i.e. supraphysiological, rates of up to 900 breaths/min at low tidal volumes (0.5–5 ml/kg). This is used in patients who have respiratory failure that has not responded to maximal, conventional ventilation, i.e. as a rescue therapy. There are four main types:

- High-frequency positive pressure ventilation
- High-frequency flow interrupted ventilation
- High-frequency jet ventilation
- High-frequency oscillation ventilation (HFOV) – this type of ventilation will be discussed in more detail as it is most commonly used.

Terminology

Frequency: Ventilation rate expressed in Hertz (Hz) – 1 Hz = 1 breath/s = 60 breaths/min

MAP: mean airway pressure (cmH$_2$O) – provides a continuous distending pressure that inflates the lung to a constant and optimal lung volume, maximising gas exchange and preventing alveolar collapse in the expiratory phase

Amplitude: delta P (ΔP), i.e. amplitude of the oscillatory wave form

Oxygenation is influenced by mean airways pressure (MAP; cmH$_2$O), F_iO_2 and amplitude to some degree. Elimination of CO_2 is influenced by amplitude (delta P), frequency and to a much smaller extent MAP. Oscillatory amplitude (difference between peak and trough pressure) directly determines tidal volumes delivered.

The actual mechanism of gaseous exchange in high frequency ventilation is not entirely understood, but a vibrating diaphragm with a constant flow of gas delivers the breaths providing active inspiration and expiration. The oscillating waveform is established around a continuous distending pressure applied to the endotracheal (ET) tube. The MAP and ΔP are significantly attenuated as they pass down the ET tube, particularly in the smaller sized ET tubes. Frequencies of 10–15Hz are most often used in neonates and infants = 600–900 breaths per minute (with higher frequencies being more lung protective).

Indications for HFOV include:

- Rescue following failure of conventional ventilation, i.e. in pulmonary hypertension of the neonate, meconium aspiration
- Air leak syndromes, i.e. pneumothorax
- To reduce barotrauma when conventional ventilator settings are high.

It is a rescue therapy for patients who have hypoxaemia and hypercarbia (but some neonatal units use it as the preferred mode of ventilation).

It is important to recognise that the HFOV can be used in many different ways and that a specific strategy should be developed on an individual patient basis when managing specific pathologies. There are several essential factors to be considered when determining the HFO strategy and these are:

- Air leak
- Pulmonary hypertension
- Impaired cardiac performance.

The clinician must also consider the current MAP on conventional ventilation, disease pathology and inflation of lung fields.

In the literature, four distinct groups of patients have been identified and strategies developed for optimal HFOV (Clark & Null 1999, Clark 1994, Kohe et al 1988).

1. Diffuse lung disease

Caused by adult respiratory distress syndrome (ARDS), respiratory distress syndrome (RDS), pulmonary haemorrhage, pneumonia (particularly Group B streptococcus).

Goal of ventilation is to improve lung inflation, compliance and ventilation/perfusion matching while avoiding barotrauma and cardiac compromise.

HFOV strategy:

- Initially MAP around 2–5 cmH$_2$O above MAP on conventional ventilator in order to maintain recruitment in the face of pressure attenuation by the ET tube (Ventre & Arnold 2004), then increase MAP in 1 cmH$_2$O increments until arterial oxygenation improves or there is a rise in central venous pressure with signs of decreased systemic blood flow, or until the chest X-ray shows normal lung inflation, or a sustained inflation manoeuvre to increase lung volume and oxygenation by re-expanding atelectatic alveoli
- Then aggressive weaning to bring the lung on to the deflation limb of the pressure volume curve (i.e. same volume at lower pressure)
- Chest X-ray required to assess degree of lung inflation
- If P_aO_2 continues to rise, wean F_iO_2 until <0.6 then wean MAP.

Initial settings IT% 0.33, F_iO_2 1.0, MAP as described above, Hz range 8–15 depending on age and size of patient. If adequate P_aCO_2 cannot be achieved with maximal power output (ΔP), decrease rate to increase tidal volume.

2. Unilateral or patchy lung involvement

For instance in meconium aspiration syndrome, focal pneumonia.

Goal of ventilation is to improve oxygenation with low MAP and to avoid lung overinflation.

HFOV strategy:

A. Pathology with air-trapping

- MAP on HFOV should be initiated at similar level as on CMV
- Amplitude should be set to achieve good chest wall movement
- Use lower range of frequency to allow more time for the delivery of larger tidal volumes distally in an effort to overcome some of the airway obstruction (i.e. 10–15 Hz).

Patients least likely to respond to HFOV are those with evidence of air-trapping and overinflation on CMV. Focal air-trapping may be accentuated by HFOV and the result may be pneumothorax and airway rupture.

B. Pathology with diffuse haze (ARDS)

- MAP above MAP on CMV
- Frequency in lower range
- Amplitude set to achieve good chest wall movement.

3. Lung hypoplasia

For instance in congenital diaphragmatic hernia, uniform pulmonary hypoplasia. These infants have small, abnormal lungs.

Goal of ventilation is to improve oxygenation at the lowest possible MAP and minimise ventilator-associated barotrauma.

HFOV strategy:

A. Uniform pulmonary hypoplasia

- MAP set at same level as CMV, then increase gradually to achieve maximum oxygen saturation. If MAP is increased by 5–6 cmH$_2$O without an increase in saturations, recheck chest X-ray for lung and vessel positioning
- Frequency 10–15 Hz
- Amplitude set to achieve **minimal** chest wall movement to minimise lung injury.

B. Non-uniform pulmonary hypoplasia (congenital diaphragmatic hernia)

- MAP started ≥CMV dependent on the contralateral lung. The MAP should be initiated in the 10–12 cmH$_2$O range and increased by 1 cmH$_2$O increments to optimise the lung volume of the unaffected lung
- Increase MAP slowly while observing cardiac function. When over-inflation occurs, the mediastinum become narrowed or may be shifted away from its optimal position and will compromise cardiac filling and output
- Frequency usually set at 10 Hz
- Amplitude set to achieve adequate chest wall movement.

4. Air leak syndromes

Goal of ventilation is use of the lowest possible ventilator settings, accept low P_aO_2 and high P_aCO_2 (with pH > 7.25)

HFOV strategy:

A. Recurrent pneumothoraces

- If the patient has poor inflation then the goal is to improve inflation by slightly increasing MAP from CMV.

Table 2.4 Management of oxygenation on HFOV considering P_aO_2 and lung compliance

If P_aO_2 is:	Lung inflation	Primary action	Secondary action
Increased	↑	↓ MAP	↓ F_iO_2
Increased	Normal	↓ F_iO_2	–
Increased	↓	↑ MAP	↓ F_iO_2
Normal	↑	↓ MAP	–
Normal	Normal	–	–
Normal	↓	↑ MAP	–
Decreased	↑	↓ MAP	↑ F_iO_2
Decreased	Normal	↑ F_iO_2	–
Decreased	↓	↑ MAP	↑ F_iO_2

Reproduced with permission from Avila et al 1994, adapted from HFO Study Group 1993.

B.   Severe air leak – with or without cysts in lungs

- MAP ⩽ MAP on CMV
- Reduce MAP by 1 cmH$_2$O increments until the target P_aO_2 is reached or chest X-ray shows normal lung inflation with signs of resolution of the air leak
- Wean MAP in preference to F_iO_2 in these patients
- Put most severely affected lung in dependent position to increase resistance to gas delivery in that lung
- Avoid hand bagging these patients if possible.

In general, once an appropriate degree of lung inflation has been achieved, a typical sequence for addressing hypercarbia would be:

- increasing delta P in increments of 3 cmH$_2$O until the power is maximised
- decrease the frequency in increments of 0.5–1.0 Hz
- partially deflating the ET tube cuff to allow the additional exit of CO$_2$ (but the decrease in MAP should be corrected by an increase in bias flow) (Ventre & Arnold 2004, VandeKieft et al 2003, Derdak et al 2002, Mehta et al 2001).

HFOV can affect cardiac output

During HFOV lung volume and pleural pressure remain relatively constant and this results in more constant and sometimes higher intrathoracic pressure that may impede venous return, and reduce cardiac output.

Patients in all groups may become candidates for ECMO so this should be considered.

Tables 2.4 and 2.5 ouline management of oxygenation and ventilation in HFOV.

Table 2.5 Management of ventilation and action to take to rectify P_aCO_2

P_aCO_2	Primary action	Secondary action
Increased	↑ oscillation amplitude	↓ frequency
Normal	–	–
Decreased	↓ oscillation amplitude	↑ frequency

Reproduced with permission from Avila et al 1994, adapted from HFO Study Group 1993.

Ventilator recording for high-frequency oscillation ventilation

Parameters that need to be set and recorded hourly or according to local hospital policy include: F_iO_2, MAP, oscillatory amplitude (ΔP) breath frequency (Hz), inspired time (IT) and flow.

If using the SLE 2000 ventilator in HFO mode, the amplitude peak inspiratory pressure, mean airways pressure, positive end expiratory pressure, inspired time, rate, patient's own rate, humidifier temperature and the fraction of inspired oxygen should be recorded hourly or according to local policy. HFO can be superimposed on to a positive pressure ventilator rate, in which case all the usual ventilator parameters will also need to be recorded.

Nitric oxide may be used in the circuit if required. The patient will still require suction and assessment of secretions (Hazinski 1992).

Consider the need for re-recruitment after suctioning.

CAPNOGRAPHY

Capnography displays a respiratory waveform representing the profile of expiratory PCO_2 over time with a numerical value for end-tidal CO_2. An infrared sensor is placed between the endotracheal tube and the ventilator tubing and this analyses the expired CO_2 at the mouth and can be used to monitor trends of alveolar ventilation and CO_2 elimination. The amount of CO_2 expired may not accurately match alveolar CO_2 because of the mixing of alveolar air with dead space. Factors that change the dead space will affect the PCO_2 and end-tidal CO_2 gradient (Laker 2003).

Capnography is useful to determine that the endotracheal tube is correctly placed and the position maintained, particularly on patient transfers. The typical shape of a capnograph waveform (Fig. 2.11) has four distinct phases:

- Phase 1: End inspiration
- Phase 2: Exhalation of dead space in trachea and large airways

Fig 2.11   Typical capnograph waveform

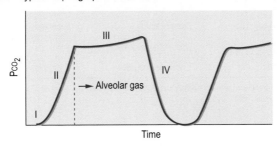

- Phase 3: Alveolar gas
- Phase 4: Early inspiration – fresh gas over sensor (Gravenstein et al 1989).

Interpreting ventilatory function using capnography – examples/trouble shooting

Oesophageal intubation/tracheal extubation (see Fig. 2.12)

This may initially show the presence of CO_2, particularly if the patient has been bag–mask ventilated but the waveform will diminish then disappear as no CO_2 will be eliminated across the sensor.

Fig 2.12   Oesophageal intubation/tracheal extubation

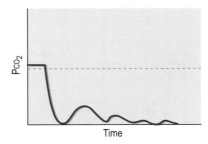

Saw tooth formation = obstructive airways, ARDS, asthma (see Fig. 2.13)

If the waveform changes from a normal waveform to this, then auscultation will be required to determine whether bronchospasm or secretions are present. Patency of endotracheal tube and ventilator tubing should also be checked (Laker 2003).

Fig 2.13 Saw tooth formation = obstructive airways

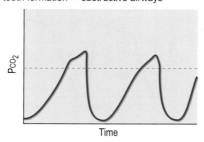

Waveform not returning to baseline (see Fig. 2.14)

This indicates rebreathing CO_2. Check expiratory valve not waterlogged or incompetent, which may be preventing expired CO_2 from escaping.

Fig 2.14 Waveform not returning to baseline

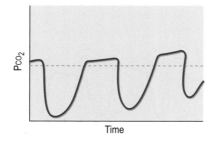

Hypoventilation (see Fig. 2.15)

Hypoventilation following bicarbonate injection, i.e. rising CO_2.

Fig 2.15   Hypoventilation

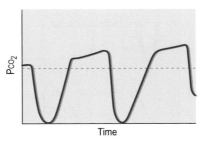

Hyperventilation (see Fig. 2.16)

Gradual fall with preservation of waveform, or decreasing cardiac output, i.e. hypovolaemic state.

Fig 2.16   Hyperventilation

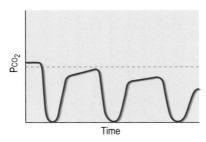

Sudden absence of any waveform (see Fig. 2.17)

Check airway disconnection, total obstruction of endotracheal tube or displaced tube, loss of cardiac output.

Fig 2.17   Sudden absence of any waveform

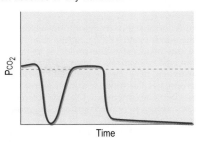

Sudden decrease in waveform amplitude (see Fig. 2.18)

Possible kinked or partially occluded endotracheal tube.

Fig 2.18   Sudden decrease in waveform amplitude

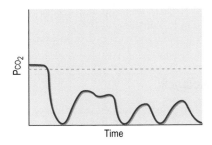

Irregular cleft in waveform (see Fig. 2.19)

This could indicate interbreathing, i.e. if paralysis is wearing off or trigger sensitivity in support mode is set too low (Laker 2003).

Fig 2.19   Irregular cleft in waveform

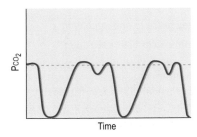

METHAEMOGLOBINAEMIA

Methaemoglobin is abnormal haemoglobin in which the iron molecule is oxidised to the ferric state (Fe^{3+}) rather than the normal ferrous state (Fe^{2+}), and this means that the molecule is incapable of binding to oxygen and can lead to cyanosis (Curry 1982, Goldfrank et al 1985). Methaemoglobinaemia may be congenital or acquired. Acquired methaemoglobinaemia is the most common form, where exposure to certain drugs or chemicals increases the rate of oxidation so that it exceeds the rate of reduction by methaemoglobin reductase systems and methaemoglobinaemia may occur.

Methaemoglobinaemia can also occur as a result of nitric oxide therapy, as nitric oxide binds to haemoglobin to produce methaemoglobin. During nitric oxide therapy, blood should be routinely tested to measure levels of methaemoglobin.

Normal methaemoglobin level <1%. Methaemoglobinaemia should be suspected (Pow 1997) if:

- cyanosis fails to respond to oxygen therapy (Goldfrank et al 1985)
- PO_2 is normal or elevated in the presence of decreased measured oxygen saturation (Goldfrank et al 1985)
- blood is brown in colour and remains dark on aeration (Mansouri 1985).

CARBOXYHAEMOGLOBIN

Carbon monoxide is a toxic, odourless gas produced by car exhausts and fires, among other causes. Carbon monoxide has a greater affinity for haemoglobin than oxygen and when bound to haemoglobin forms carboxyhaemoglobin. This impairs oxygen transport, produces decreased oxygen delivery and tissue hypoxia, and can result in metabolic acidosis if carbon monoxide levels are high. Levels of carboxyhaemoglobin above 60% are often fatal (Hazinski 1992).

ORAL INTUBATION

Step-by-step guide to oral intubation

Consider three steps before starting:

- Can you bag–mask ventilate adequately?
- Can you intubate?
- Do you have a fall-back, e.g. laryngeal mask, if unable to intubate?

Assess whether the child is likely to have a difficult airway, e.g.:

- Pierre Robin's syndrome

- Down's syndrome
- Goldenhar's syndrome
- Mucopolysaccharidosis – Hunter's, Hurler's syndromes
- Cleft palate
- Patients with dysmorphic features, large tongue, small chin
- Patients with facial burns, ARDS.

This is not a definitive list – just examples.

Call for expert assistance in anticipation rather than as an emergency.

- Prepare all equipment prior to starting intubation – see Box 2.3
- Ensure oxygen and suction are to hand and in working order
- Monitor heart rate and oxygen saturations if possible, as the process of intubation may induce bradycardia and hypoxia
- Ensure monitoring is audible
- If not an emergency situation, pass a nasogastric tube prior to intubation
- Position patient and preoxygenate in 100% oxygen for a few minutes. NB. Do not preoxygenate if baby has hypoplastic left heart syndrome, as this will destabilise him/her
- Give drugs/anaesthetic agents if required, e.g. ketamine, atracurium, etc. Only give muscle relaxant once the patient is adequately anaesthetised and you know you can ventilate adequately using a mask and rebreathe bag – see Box 2.4 Common intubation drugs

---

Box 2.3 Equipment required for oral intubation

- Laryngoscope and appropriate blade:
  - Neonate – small, straight blade
  - Young child – small, curved blade
  - Older child – large, curved blade
- Magill's forceps, appropriate size
- Yankauer sucker and suction – to gauge appropriate size: size of ET tube used ×2 = French gauge of catheter required
- Rebreathing circuit or Ambu bag – appropriate size
- Oxygen supply
- Introducer stylet: S, M or L and bougie
- Endotracheal tube
  - Correct size+
  - spare tube of same size+
  - spare tube one size smaller
- Catheter mount connector attaches from end of endotracheal tube to rebreathe or ventilator circuit
- Nasogastric tube
- Assorted tapes if oral intubation+
  - Duoderm to protect skin
- Drugs prior to intubation according to prescription
- Drugs for resuscitation and fluids in unstable patient.

> **Box 2.4   Common drug doses used for intubation (check local policy)**
>
> Ketamine 1–2 mg/kg
> Rocuronium 0.6 mg/kg
> Atracurium 0.3–0.6 mg/kg
> Morphine 0.1 mg/kg
> Etomidate 0.3 mg/kg
> Thiopentone 2–7 mg/kg

- Doctor will use laryngoscope to visualise vocal cords and use Yankauer sucker to clear airway, then will pass oral endotracheal tube – see Box 2.5 for appropriate ETT size
- Resume ventilation
- Cut all tapes as required if not cut already, i.e. in emergency situation
  - Two thin Granuflex strips to protect the cheeks from mouth to ear
  - Two strips of Elastoplast or similar tape cut as trouser legs
  - Other appropriate tapes if other methods of securing ET tube are used, e.g. Melbourne strapping or 'trouser leg' tapes to stick to face and tube
- If a nasal tube is required, remove oral tube on doctor's request – then, when nasal tube in position, connect to catheter mount connection or other appropriate connector and resume ventilation
- Observe and auscultate chest for equal, bilateral chest movement and sounds to determine correct placement of ET tube and connect to end tidal CO_2 monitor to confirm end-tidal trace and tracheal intubation
- If so, secure tube with tapes
- Chest X-ray as soon as possible to reconfirm position. Table 2.6 lists endotracheal sizes and lengths
- Preoxygenate prior to suctioning

Selection of endotracheal tube

> **Box 2.5   Formula for calculating ET tube requirements**
>
> Endotracheal tube size (mm) $= \dfrac{\text{Age (years)}}{4} + 4$
>
> Oral length (cm) $= \dfrac{\text{Age (years)}}{2} + 12$
>
> Nasal length (cm) $= \dfrac{\text{Age (years)}}{2} + 15$

Table 2.6 Endotracheal tube – sizes and lengths

Age	Weight (kg)	Internal diameter (mm)	Length	
			At lips (cm)	At nose (cm)
Newborn	1–3	3.0	6–8.5	7.5–10.5
Newborn	3.5	3.5	9	11
3 months	6	3.5	10	12
1 year	10	4.0	11	14
2 years	12	4.5	12	15
3 years	14	4.5	13	16
4 years	16	5.0	14	17
6 years	20	5.5	15	19
8 years	24	6.0	16	20
10 years	30	6.5	17	21
12 years	38	7.0	18	22
14 years	50	7.5	19	23

Below 8 years of age, an uncuffed tube is used, as the larynx at the level of the cricoid cartilage is the narrowest point and will form a natural seal. After the age of 8 years, the cricoid larynx becomes wider and a cuff may be required to prevent air leakage at this level.
Source: reproduced with permission from Shann 2003.

USE OF INHALED NITRIC OXIDE

Nitric oxide (NO) is a powerful pulmonary vasodilator that has specific action and does not cause systemic hypotension. It can be used in patients who have reversible pulmonary hypertension and/or ventilation perfusion mismatch, e.g. neonates with persistent pulmonary hypertension of the neonate, children with congenital heart disease and pulmonary hypertension, or children with acute respiratory distress syndrome (ARDS).

Nitric oxide must be prescribed. A common starting dose of nitric oxide would be 1–5 parts per million and this may be increased as prescribed to a top therapeutic dose of around 20 parts per million; however, regulation of this is sometimes difficult.

In addition to normal observations and blood tests, when using nitric oxide, blood levels of nitrogen dioxide (NO_2) and methaemoglobin should be tested and both, ideally, should be below 1%. (Methaemoglobin levels should be taken 12–24-hourly.)

NO cylinders should be checked regularly to ensure that they do not run out. Infants and children can become very dependent on NO and the rebound effect if the NO supply failed could be fatal.

Analysers must be used to measure NO and NO_2 concentrations.

Scavenger systems can be used, i.e. a charcoal filter can be placed on the exhaust of the ventilator, which gets rid of NO and NO_2 from the circuit.

A circuit should be set up to hand-ventilate the child with NO if s/he is particularly sensitive to it.

Closed-circuit suction should be considered if the child is very sensitive to NO. If normal suction is used, consider giving extra breaths using the manual breath button on the ventilator prior to suction. Record NO concentration hourly on the ITU chart.

REFERENCES

Avila K, Mazza L, Morgan-Trujillo L 1994 High frequency oscillatory ventilation: a nursing approach to bedside care. Neonat Netw 13(5): 23–30

British Thoracic Society Standards of Care Committee 2002 Non-invasive ventilation in acute respiratory failure. Thorax 57: 192–211

Clark RH et al, 1994 Prospective, randomised comparison of HFO and conventional ventilation in candidates for ECMO. J Pediatr 124: 447–454

Clark RH, Null DM 1999 High frequency oscillation ventilation: clinical management strategies. Critical Care Review. SensorMedics Corporation, Yorba Linda, CA

Corne J, Carroll M, Brown I, Delany D 2002 Chest X-ray made easy. 2nd edn. Churchill Livingstone, London

Curry S 1982 Methaemoglobinaemia. Ann Emerg Med 11: 214–221

Derdak S, Mehta S, Stewart TE et al 2002 High-frequency oscillatory ventilation for acute respiratory distress syndrome in adults: a randomised controlled trial. Am J Respir Crit Care Med 166: 801–808

Fort P, Farmer C, Westerman J et al 1997 High-frequency oscillatory ventilation for adult respiratory distress syndrome – a pilot study. Crit Care Med 25: 937–947

Goldfrank LR, Price D, Kirstein RH 1985 Goldfrank's toxicological emergencies, 3rd edn. Appleton & Lange, Norwalk, CT

Gravenstein JS, Paulus D, Hayes TJ 1989 Capnography in clinical practice. Butterworth Publishers, Stoneham, MA

Hazinski M F (ed) 1992 Nursing care of the critically ill child, 2nd edn. Mosby Year Book, St Louis, MO

HFO Study Group 1993 Randomised study of high frequency oscillation ventilation in infants with severe respiratory distress syndrome. J Pediatr 122: 609–619

Hinds C J, Watson D 1996 Intensive care, 2nd edn. W B Saunders, London

Kohe D et al 1988 High frequency oscillation in the rescue of infants with persistent pulmonary hypertension. Crit Care Med 16, 510–6

Laker S 2003 Part 2: Capnography in respiratory monitoring. In Flight Nursing News, Autumn. Royal College of Nursing, London

Mansouri A 1985 Review: methaemoglobinaemia. Am J Med Sci 289: 200–208

Medivent Ltd 2002 RTX Operator's Manual. Medivent Ltd, Lucan, Co. Dublin

Mehta S, Lapinsky SE, Hallett DC et al 2001. Prospective trial of high frequency oscillation in adults with acute respiratory distress syndrome. Crit Care Med 29: 1360–1369

Miller MJ, Martin RJ, Carlo WA et al 1985 Oral breathing in newborn infants. J Pediatr 107: 465

Miller MJ, Carlo WA, Strohl KP et al 1986 Effect of maturation on oral breathing in sleeping premature infants. J Pediatr 109: 515–519

Pow J 1997 Methaemoglobinaemia: an unusual blue boy. Paediatr Nurs 9(10): 24–25

Resuscitation Council (UK) 2004 Acid–base balance: interpreting arterial blood gases. Advanced Life Support Manual, Appendix. Resuscitation Council (UK), London, p 142

Schelvan C, Copeman A, Young J, Davis J 2002 Paediatric Radiology for MRCPH/FRCR. Royal Society of Medicine, London

Shann F 2003 Drug doses, 12th edn. Intensive Care Unit, Royal Children's Hospital, Parkville, Victoria

Siemens Medical Engineering 1993 System SV300. Life Support Systems, Sweden

Taylor M B, Whitwam J G 1986 The current status of pulse oximetry. Anaesthesia 41: 943–949

Tortora G J, Anagnostakos N P 1984 Principles of anatomy and physiology, 4th edn. Harper, Sydney, NSW

VandeKieft M, Dorsey D et al 2003 Effects of endotracheal cuff leak on gas flow patterns in a mechanical lung model during high frequency oscillatory ventilation. Am J Respir Crit Care Med A178

Ventre KM, Arnold JH 2004 High frequency oscillatory ventilation in acute respiratory failure. Paediatr Respir Rev 5: 323–332

VIASYS Healthcare Clinical Training Book: The Infant Flow System

Useful websites

www.eme-med.co.uk
www.mediventintl.com
www.ViasysCriticalCare.com

FETAL CIRCULATION

The fetal circulation differs anatomically and physiologically from the postnatal circulation:

- Blood oxygenation takes place in the placenta
- The fetus is relatively hypoxaemic, with O_2 saturation of 60–70%
- Tissue hypoxia does not occur because fetal cardiac output is so high – approx. 400–500 ml/kg/min (Hazinski 1992) – and because fetal haemoglobin has a high oxygen-carrying capacity
- The fetal circulation is designed to deliver the best oxygenated blood to the fetal brain and allow blood to be diverted away from the pulmonary circulation
- Fetal systemic vascular resistance (SVR) is low – nearly half of all descending aortic blood flow enters the placenta, which provides little resistance to blood flow
- Fetal pulmonary vascular resistance (PVR) is very high – the lungs are fluid-filled and the resultant alveolar hypoxia contributes to intense pulmonary vasoconstriction. This results in blood flowing away from the lungs towards the low resistance of the placenta (Fig. 3.1)
- Oxygenated blood enters the fetus via the umbilical vein $\rightarrow$ ductus venosus, bypassing the hepatic circulation, which flows into the inferior vena cava (IVC)
- The blood enters the right atrium and flows across the foramen ovale into the left atrium
- The blood then enters the left ventricle $\rightarrow$ ascending aorta $\rightarrow$ perfuses the head and upper extremities
- The lower part of the fetal body is perfused by a small amount of the well oxygenated blood flowing from the ascending aorta and a proportionately large amount of poorly oxygenated blood from the patent ductus arteriosus (PDA)
- Venous blood from the head and upper extremities returns via the SVC $\rightarrow$ right atrium $\rightarrow$ right ventricle $\rightarrow$ pulmonary artery
- Because of the high PVR this blood flows $\rightarrow$ PDA $\rightarrow$ ascending aorta as above. Much of this flow will then return to the placenta via the umbilical arteries.

Fig 3.1 Blood flow through the fetal circulation (with permission from Williams & Asquith 2000)

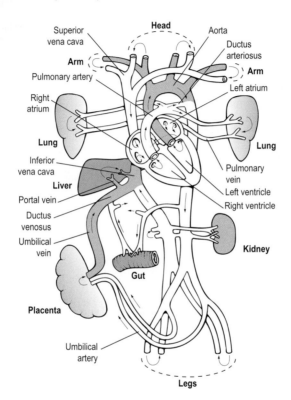

Changes in the fetal circulation at birth

- When the baby starts breathing, the PVR falls; the increase in O_2 and negative intrathoracic pressure divert blood to the lungs and away from the PDA, causing it to constrict and subsequently close
- Because of increased pulmonary blood flow, pressure in the left atrium is increased and raised above that of the right atrium, causing the flap valve of the patent foramen ovale to close (it can be reopened if necessary by, for example, balloon septostomy)
- When the umbilical cord is clamped, the ductus venosus constricts and closes.

THE NORMAL HEART

- Venous blood enters the right atrium via the superior vena cava (SVC) – from the head and the upper body – and the IVC – from the lower body
- Blood flows from the right atrium through a tricuspid valve into the right ventricle
- The right ventricle pumps the blood through the pulmonary valve into the pulmonary artery and then to the lungs to be oxygenated. The main trunk of the pulmonary artery divides into two – right and left pulmonary arteries – to supply each lung separately
- From the lungs the oxygenated blood flows to the left atrium via the pulmonary veins
- From the left atrium the blood flows into the left ventricle through the mitral valve
- The left ventricle pumps the oxygenated blood through the aortic valve into the ascending aorta and from there to the systemic circulation (Fig. 3.2).

Fig 3.2   Blood flow through the normal heart (with permission from Wilson 1987)

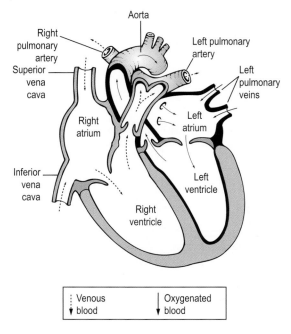

CLASSIFICATION OF CONGENITAL HEART DISEASE

When planning the care and management of children with congenital heart disease, it may be useful to categorise defects in terms of alteration to blood flow. Most cardiac defects fall into one of four categories (Fig. 3.3):

Increased pulmonary flow

- Patent ductus arteriosis (PDA)
- Atrial septal defect (ASD)
- Ventricular septal defect (VSD)
- Atrioventricular septal defect (AVSD)

Decreased pulmonary flow

- Pulmonary stenosis
- Pulmonary atresia
- Fallot's tetralogy
- Tricuspid atresia

Decreased systemic flow

- Coarctation of aorta
- Aortic stenosis
- Interrupted aortic arch
- Hypoplastic left heart syndrome (HLHS)

Fig 3.3   Classification of congenital heart disease

Increased pulmonary flow	Decreased systemic flow
PDA ASD VSD AVSD	Coarctation of aorta Aortic stenosis Interrupted aortic arch HLHS
Decreased pulmonary flow	Altered circulation
Pulmonary stenosis Pulmonary atresia Fallot's tetralogy Tricuspid atresia	TGA Truncus arteriosis TAPVD Double outlet right ventricle (DORV)

Altered circulation

- Transposition of the great arteries (TGA)
- Truncus arteriosus
- Total anomalous pulmonary venous drainage (TAPVD)
- Double outlet right ventricle

Defects with increased pulmonary blood flow

Patent ductus arteriosis

Persistence of this duct beyond the perinatal period – usually closes spontaneously within hours of birth.

Effect: Blood flows from the aorta through the PDA to the pulmonary artery – therefore there is increased flow to the lungs.

Management: Closed by cardiac catheter 'umbrella' procedure or surgically ligated – thoracotomy approach. In the preterm infant, indomethacin (prostaglandin synthetase inhibitor) may be used to close the PDA.

> With some complex cardiac defects, it is imperative that the ductus arteriosus is kept patent in order to maintain pulmonary blood flow (e.g. pulmonary atresia) or systemic blood flow (e.g. coarctation of aorta/hypoplastic left heart). A prostaglandin E_2 infusion will be set up in order to maintain a PDA (see Ch. 9).

Post-op: Subacute bacterial endocarditis (SBE) prophylaxis for 6 months after successful surgery

Atrial septal defect

A hole in the atrial septum.

Effect: Blood shunts left $\rightarrow$ right.

Management: Closed by cardiac catheter 'umbrella' procedure or surgically – patch repair involving bypass surgery.

Post-op: Possibility of atrial arrhythmias.

Ventricular septal defect

A hole in the ventricular septum.

Effect: Blood shunts left $\rightarrow$ right; therefore if large, greatly increased flow to lungs. NB. If pulmonary stenosis is present, flow may be right $\rightarrow$ left.

Management:

- Palliative – pulmonary artery (PA) banding to restrict flow to the lungs
- Corrective – patch repair to VSD and remove PA band, involving bypass surgery. If small, some centres may close VSD via cardiac catheter 'umbrella' procedure.

Post-op: Possibility of residual leak across patch, when SBE prophylaxis should be observed.

Atrioventricular septal defect

Openings in both the atrial and ventricular septa.

Effect: Mixing of oxygenated and deoxygenated blood at both levels. May result in atrioventricular valve regurgitation, congestive cardiac failure and left $\rightarrow$ right shunt with pulmonary hypertension.

Management:

- Palliative – pulmonary artery banding to reduce flow to the lungs
- Corrective – bypass surgery to perform patch closures to ASD and VSD and reconstruct clefts of atrioventricular valves if necessary.

Post-op: Possibility of arrhythmias (particularly supraventricular tachycardia (SVT)), degree of cardiac failure due to valve incompetence, pulmonary hypertension. SBE prophylaxis usually indicated.

Defects with decreased pulmonary blood flow

Pulmonary stenosis

Narrowing of the entrance to the pulmonary artery due to either pulmonary valve or pulmonary outflow tract obstruction.

Effect: Reduced blood flow to the lungs. Usually asymptomatic with mild stenosis. Neonates with critical pulmonary stenosis are cyanotic and tachypnoeic.

Management: For neonates with critical pulmonary stenosis and cyanosis, a prostaglandin E_2 infusion to reopen the ductus should be started. Stenosed area widened by cardiac catheter technique – inflated end passed through narrowed artery – or surgical correction – patch widening of the right ventricular outflow tract (RVOT). Valvotomy if the valve is the cause.

Post-op: SBE may be indicated.

Pulmonary atresia

An atretic pulmonary valve, resulting from its failure to develop.

Effect: The interventricular septum is intact – no blood flow from the right ventricle (RV) to the lungs. The neonate is dependent on other defects (ASD, PDA) for survival. The size of the right ventricle is variable and related to survival. There is severe and progressive cyanosis from birth.

Management:

- Palliative Maintain PDA with prostaglandin E_2 infusion. Balloon atrial septostomy may be indicated to improve right to left atrial shunting of blood in patients with right ventricular sinusoids (irregular channels in which blood vessels anastomose)
- Correction Initial and follow up surgical procedures. Three types of surgical decision depending on size of right ventricle and the presence or absence of right ventricular sinusoids or coronary artery anomalies
- If right ventricle is adequate in size for future growth, establish connection between right ventricle and main PA (transannular patch or closed transpulmonary valvotomy) in preparation for a two-ventricle repair. A systemic–pulmonary shunt is also performed at the same time. Alternatively, use of laser-wire and radiofrequency assisted valvotomy plus balloon dilatation of the pulmonary annulus has been shown to be safer and more efficacious
- For monopartite right ventricle and sinusoids, a systemic–pulmonary shunt without the RV outflow patch is recommended as decompression of the RV (by valvotomy or an outflow patch) may reverse coronary flow into the RV, producing myocardial ischaemia. A Fontan operation can be performed later
- If coronary anomalies identified by aortogram, the sinusoids are left alone. If no coronary artery anomalies are identified, either sinusoidal ligation or closure of the tricuspid valve (thromboexclusion of the RV) may be performed. This increases suitability for eventual Fontan.

Follow-up procedures:

- For those who received the RVOT patch and a systemic–pulmonary shunt and show evidence of RV cavity growth, the shunt is closed if the patient tolerates balloon occlusion of the shunt during cardiac catheterisation
- For those who received a closed pulmonary valvotomy and a systemic–pulmonary shunt and who have a large enough RV, a RVOT reconstruction and closure of ASD and shunt are performed
- For those who continue to have hypoplasia of the RV and tricuspid valve annulus, a Fontan-type operation is performed later
- An additional shunt operation may be necessary in patients on whom none of the above procedures can be performed.

Post-op: Most patients require close follow-up as none of the surgical procedures are curative. SBE prophylaxis if indicated.

Fallot's tetralogy (Fig. 3.4)

Four elements:

- VSD
- Pulmonary stenosis
- Overriding aorta
- Right ventricular hypertrophy.

Effect: Degree of cyanosis depends on size of VSD and degree of pulmonary stenosis, which affect direction of blood shunting through VSD.
  Hypoxic 'spells' may occur, characterised by:

- paroxysm of hyperpnoea (rapid and deep respiration)
- irritability and prolonged crying
- increasing cyanosis
- decreased intensity of the heart murmur.

A severe spell may lead to limpness, convulsions, cerebrovascular accident or even death. Management is aimed at breaking the vicious cycle

Fig 3.4 Blood flow through the heart with Fallot's tetralogy (adapted with permission from Whaley & Wong 1991)

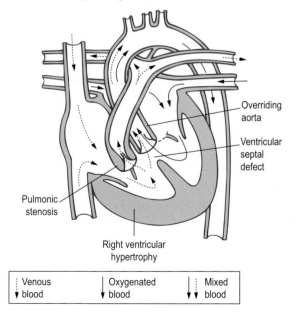

Overriding aorta

Ventricular septal defect

Pulmonic stenosis

Right ventricular hypertrophy

| ┊ Venous
▼ blood | │ Oxygenated
▼ blood | ┊ │ Mixed
▼ ▼ blood |

and includes positioning, IV morphine/ketamine, reducing acidosis and administering O_2.

Management:

- Palliative If pulmonary stenosis is severe, BT shunt (anastomosis between the subclavian artery and ipsilateral pulmonary artery) prior to total correction to improve pulmonary blood flow
- Total correction Bypass surgery involving VSD patch closure and patch widening of RVOT.

Post-op: Possibility of arrhythmias, particularly ventricular tachycardia, and pulmonary hypertension. May require additional fluid to optimise preload because of right ventricular hypertrophy. Varying levels of activity limitation may be indicated. SBE prophylaxis may be indicated.

Tricuspid atresia

An atretic tricuspid valve resulting from its failure to develop.

Effect: No blood flow from right atrium to right ventricle and therefore to the lungs. The neonate is dependent on other defects (e.g. PDA, ASD, VSD) for survival: TGA may also be present. Severe cyanosis and tachypnea are usual.

Management:

- Palliative Maintain PDA with prostaglandin E_2 infusion and BT or Waterston shunt (anastomosis between the ascending aorta and right pulmonary artery) to ensure blood flow to lungs
- Correction Stage 1, bidirectional Glenn shunt – SVC to right pulmonary artery anastomosis with blood flow to both lungs. Stage 2, Fontan procedure – baffle (tunnel) of IVC flow through right atrium connecting directly to right pulmonary artery where SVC is also directly connected. A fenestration (hole) may be present in the baffle, allowing some escape into the right atrium if the pressure in the baffle becomes high.

Post–op: For Glenn and Fontan procedures, extubate early (positive pressure ventilation impedes venous drainage). Possibility of pleural effusions due to high right-sided venous pressure. May need to be excluded from competitive sports and receive SBE prophylaxis.

Defects with decreased systemic blood flow

Coarctation of aorta

Severe narrowing of a segment of the aorta.
 This may be:

- Preductal Narrowing proximal to ductus arteriosus. PDA allows blood to shunt from the pulmonary artery to descending aorta

- Postductal Narrowing distal to ductus arteriosus. PDA allows blood to shunt from aorta to pulmonary artery. Collateral circulation may supply blood from the subclavian arteries to the descending aorta
- Periductal Narrowing located at level of ductus arteriosus. Bidirectional shunting through the PDA may occur (proximal aorta → PDA; PDA → distal aorta).

Effect: Reduction in circulatory blood flow, signs of congestive heart failure and renal failure, which may lead to general circulatory shock.

Management: Surgical correction (not usually requiring bypass) in infancy if symptomatic − end-to-end anastomosis or subclavian flap repair (subclavian artery ligated so unable to obtain cuff BP in that arm). NB. There is a risk of necrotising enterocolitis because of decreased mesenteric blood flow. If coarctation of aorta is suspected, perform four-limb cuff BP in order to make comparisons.

Post-op: Possibility of hypertension − infusion of vasodilator drugs, e.g. glyceryl trinitrate (GTN) may be required. Necrotising enterocolitis/acute renal failure may develop, depending on the degree to which the blood supply was compromised. Re-coarctation may occur. SBE prophylaxis may be indicated.

Aortic stenosis

Obstruction to the blood flow between the left ventricle and the aorta caused by stenosis (narrowing) of the aortic valve at various locations:

- Valvular (most common) A bicuspid rather than tricuspid aortic valve is the most common form of aortic stenosis
- Subvalvular Muscular obstruction below the aortic valve; may be due to long, tunnel-like narrowing of the left ventricular outflow tract or another type of subvalvular stenosis, idiopathic hypertrophic sub-aortic stenosis (IHSS), which is a primary disorder of the heart muscle (cardiomyopathy)
- Supravalvular Aortic narrowing immediately above the valve, often associated with Williams' syndrome (mental retardation, characteristic 'elfin face' and pulmonary stenosis).

Effect: Newborn infants with critical aortic stenosis may develop congestive heart failure, with a clinical picture resembling sepsis with low cardiac output. Left ventricular hypertrophy may develop if the stenosis is severe. A poststenotic dilatation of the ascending aorta develops with valvular aortic stenosis. Aortic regurgitation usually develops in subaortic aortic stenosis.

Management:

- Palliative In critically ill infants and children with congestive heart failure, O_2, diuretics and inotropes, possibly with prostaglandin infusion are indicated, with urgent need for surgery

- Balloon valvuloplasty may be performed at cardiac catheterisation
- Exercise restriction in children with moderate–severe form, good oral hygiene and SBE prophylaxis are important
- Surgical Closed aortic valvotomy using calibrated dilators or balloon catheter without cardiac bypass, or the following procedures may be performed under cardiac bypass
- Artificial valve replacement Replacement with pulmonary valve auto-graft (Ross procedure – see below); valve replacement following aortic root enlargement (Konno procedure) for tunnel-like narrowing; excision of the membrane for discrete subvalvular stenosis; widening of the stenotic area using a diamond-shaped fabric patch for discrete supravalvular stenosis.

Post-op: Restriction from competitive sports recommended with children with moderate residual aortic stenosis/regurgitation. SBE prophylaxis if indicated. Recurrence of discrete recurrent subaortic stenosis is frequent following surgical resection of the membrane.

Ross procedure: The Ross procedure is an aortic valve replacement in which the patient's own pulmonary valve is transplanted to the aortic valve position and the pulmonary valve is replaced with a homograft. An advantage for children is that the replaced aortic valve retains growth potential and does not require anticoagulation therapy.

Interrupted aortic arch

Interrupted is the absence or discontinuation of a portion of the aortic arch. There are three types, classified according to the site of the interruption:

- Type A Interruption occurs just beyond the left subclavian artery – approx. 30–40% reported cases
- Type B Interruption occurs between the left carotid artery and the left subclavian artery: most common – approx. 53% reported cases
- Type C Interruption occurs between innominate artery and left carotid artery – least common: approx. 4% reported cases (Cincinnati Childrens Hospital Medical Center 2004)

Effect: PDA and VSD are almost always associated with this defect; patients with type B often have DiGeorge's syndrome; bicuspid aortic valve, mitral valve deformity, persistent truncus arteriosis or subaortic stenosis may be present.

Infants with PDA may appear asymptomatic. If VSD present L → R shunting causes increased blood flow to the lungs and congestive heart failure. As the PDA closes, respiratory distress, cyanosis and circulatory shock develop.

Management:

- Palliative Prostaglandin E_2 infusion, intubation and ventilation, ascertain serum calcium and test for DiGeorge syndrome (i.e. chromosomal analysis for 22q deletion)

- Corrective Surgical repair of interruption (primary anastomosis, vascular graft) and closure of a simple VSD are recommended if possible. If associated with complex defects, repair of the interruption and PA banding are performed initially with complete repair later.

Hypoplastic left heart syndrome (Fig. 3.5)

A collection of complex defects on the left side of the heart:

- Underdeveloped left ventricle
- Mitral valve stenosis/atresia
- Hypoplastic ascending aorta and aortic arch
- Aortic stenosis/atresia.

Effect: Infant is reliant on PDA for systemic blood flow and patent foramen ovale (PFO) for mixing of blood at atrial level. Neonates present in hypotensive shock if ductus closure occurs, the inadequate systemic

Fig 3.5   Blood flow through the heart in hypoplastic left heart syndrome (adapted with permission from Whaley & Wong 1991)

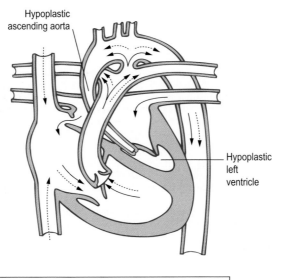

Hypoplastic ascending aorta

Hypoplastic left ventricle

⋮ Venous ▼ blood	┊ Oxygenated ▼ blood	⋮┊ Mixed ▼▼ blood

blood flow causing a profound metabolic acidosis. Fatal without surgical intervention.

Management

Three options:

- The infant is allowed to die if parents do not wish to proceed with surgery – if identified antenatally, counselling and termination may be offered
- Transplantation (not generally considered in the UK)
- Surgery in three stages – the Norwood procedure, which is outlined here.

Pre-op:

- Prostaglandin E_2 infusion to maintain PDA and therefore adequate systemic perfusion
- Aim for S_aO_2 75–85% to balance lungs versus systemic blood flow by using room air
- May need to intubate and ventilate – keeping P_{CO_2} at 5–6 kPa will increase pulmonary vascular resistance and help to keep S_aO_2 within desired range
- Correct acidosis

 If the infant desaturates, increase F_iO_2, but if it is necessary to bag the infant, bag in **air**; remembering that O_2 is a pulmonary vasodilator, therefore use air to avoid unnecessary pulmonary vascular vasodilatation and subsequent pulmonary overcirculation. Consider also the effect of CO_2 (pulmonary vasoconstriction); hyperventilation will lower the CO_2 and again may cause pulmonary overcirculation.

Stage 1 – Norwood procedure (Fig. 3.6):

- Division of main pulmonary artery and closure of distal stump
- Modified right BT shunt between subclavian artery and right pulmonary artery to provide pulmonary blood flow
- PDA is ligated and atrial septum excised to allow mixing of blood across atria
- Construction of new aortic arch between the main pulmonary artery and ascending aorta and arch.

Post-op: Anticoagulation to maintain the BT shunt. Manipulate P_{CO_2} to balance the pulmonary vs systemic blood flow, e.g. keep P_{CO_2} at 5–6 kPa and aim for S_aO_2 75–85%. (Each centre will have its own protocols.)

Fig 3.6 Norwood procedure

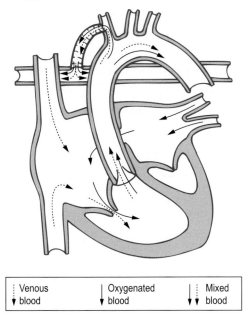

| ⁝ Venous | ▎Oxygenated | ⁝▎ Mixed |
| ▼ blood | ▼ blood | ▼▼ blood |

Stage 1 – Sano shunt: Pulmonary overcirculation through a systemic-pulmonary shunt (as above) has been documented as one of the major causes of early death after the Norwood procedure (Sano et al 2003). In order to avoid this a right ventricle → pulmonary shunt known as the Sano shunt has been employed in the first stage of palliation surgery. The important advantage of the Sano shunt is that flow occurs only during systole, with no competition between pulmonary and coronary blood flow during diastole as is the case with the Blalock shunt. This is the most likely explanation for the much improved stability of neonates which is seen following a Sano shunt (Jonas 2003).

• Division of proximal main pulmonary artery and closure of distal main pulmonary artery
• PTFE (Gore-Tex®) tube and cuff anastomosed to the distal end of the main pulmonary artery
• Anastomosis of descending aorta to posterior wall of aortic arch. Entire aortic arch and ascending aorta reconstructed by direct anastomosis of

Fig 3.7   RV–PA shunt (with permission from Sano et al 2003)

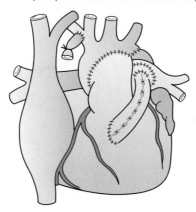

proximal main pulmonary artery. Small right ventriculotomy made in outflow tract for proximal anastomosis of RV–PA shunt (Fig. 3.7)

- After completion of aortic reconstruction and atrial septectomy, proximal anastomosis of the RV–PA shunt was performed with the heart beating.

Post-op: Similar principles to post-op management of previous stage 1 Norwood except that pulmonary versus systemic balance of circulation is more stable, as described above, and management is therefore reported to be more 'routine' (Jonas 2003).

Stage 1 – Hybrid procedure:

- Banding of pulmonary arteries to limit blood flow to lungs
- Stent to ductus arteriosis to maintain patency.

An advantage of this procedure is that bypass is not required.

Post op: Potential problem of stent migration.

Stage 2 – Hemi-Fontan/bidirectional Glenn shunt:

- Performed at age of 3–6 months
- SVC → right atrium or pulmonary artery anastomosis with intra-atrial baffle
- Aim is to separate pulmonary/systemic flow. (Fig. 3.8)

Fig 3.8   Hemi-Fontan/bidirectional Glenn shunt

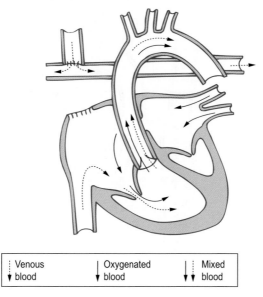

: Venous		Oxygenated	:: Mixed
▼ blood	▼ blood	▼▼ blood

Post-op: Refer to management of Glenn shunt.

Stage 3 – Modified Fontan: Performed at age of 3–5 years (Fig. 3.9).

Post-op: Refer to management of Fontan procedure. Long-term follow-up.

Altered circulation

Transposition of the great arteries

The aorta arises from the right ventricle and the pulmonary artery from the left ventricle (Fig. 3.10).

Effect: Systemic venous blood returns to the systemic arterial circulation and pulmonary – oxygenated – blood returns to the pulmonary circulation. Survival is impossible unless an additional defect (e.g. PFO, PDA, VSD) is present to allow mixing of oxygenated and deoxygenated blood.

Fig 3.9   Modified Fontan procedure

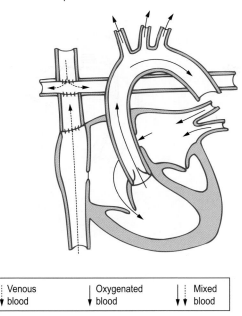

| :   Venous | | Oxygenated | : :   Mixed |
| ▼ blood | ▼ blood | ▼ ▼ blood |

Management: Prostaglandin E_2 infusion to maintain PDA. Balloon atrial septostomy via cardiac catheterisation to improve mixing of blood if septum intact. Surgical correction is usually a Jatene (switch) procedure in the neonatal period, in which the pulmonary artery and aorta are transposed and the coronary arteries are reimplanted into the aorta in its new location.

Post-op: Possibility of coronary artery obstruction causing myocardial ischaemia/infarction/left ventricular dysfunction, when limitation of activity may be indicated. SBE prophylaxis may be indicated.

 Pre-op, if it is necessary to bag the infant use **air** if required because of the effect this will have on systemic flow (as discussed under HLHS).

Rastelli operation: This surgery is indicated for patients with TGA, VSD and pulmonary stenosis. It comprises a RV to PA connection (Fig. 3.11).

Fig 3.10   Blood flow through the heart with transposition of the great arteries (adapted with permission from Whaley & Wong 1991)

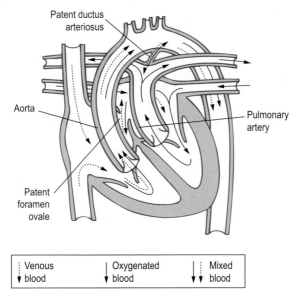

| Venous : blood | Oxygenated blood | Mixed : blood |

Fig 3.11   Rastelli operation. A. The PA is divided from the LV, and the cardiac end is oversewn (arrow). B. An intracardiac tunnel (arrow) is placed between the large VSD and the aorta. C. The RV is connected to the divided PA by an aortic homograft or a valve-bearing prosthetic conduit (redrawn with permission from Park 2003)

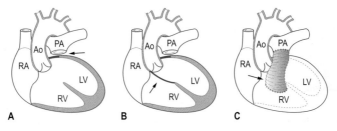

A   B   C

Fig 3.12 Damus–Kaye–Stansel operation. A. Incision made in the ascending aorta. B. Anastomosis of the proximal main PA end to side of the ascending aorta using Dacron tube or Gore-Tex. This will direct left ventricular blood flow to the aorta. The aortic valve is either closed or left unclosed. C. The VSD is closed by a right ventricular ventriculotomy and a valved conduit is placed between the right ventricle and distal PA. This channel will carry right ventricular blood flow to the PA (redrawn with permission from Park 2003)

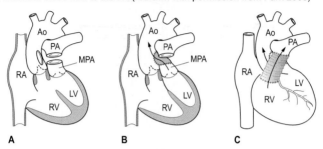

A   **B**   **C**

Fig 3.13 Congenitally corrected TGA (redrawn with permission from Park 2003)

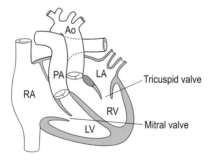

Damus–Kaye–Stansel operation: This surgery is indicated for patients with TGA, VSD and subaortic stenosis. It comprises transection of the main PA near its bifurcation (Fig. 3.12).

Congenitally corrected TGA

The atrial arrangement is normal, i.e. the right atrium (RA) is on the right of the left atrium (LA) (Fig. 3.13). However:

- The RA empties into the anatomical left ventricle (LV) (identified as such by the presence of the mitral rather than tricuspid valve)

- The LA empties into the anatomical right ventricle (RV) (identified as such by the presence of the tricuspid rather than mitral valve)
- The great arteries are transposed, with the aorta arising from the RV and the PA arising from the LV. The aorta lies to the left of and anterior to the PA
- The final result is a functional correction – oxygenated blood entering the LA flows to the anatomic RV and then out via the aorta.

Effect: Theoretically, no functional abnormalities exist, but most cases are complicated by associated defects: VSD with/without pyloric stenosis (PS) resulting in cyanosis; regurgitation of the systemic AV (tricuspid) valve; varying degrees of heart block; SVT.

Management:

- Palliative Treatment of congestive heart failure and arrhythmias; SBE prophylaxis if indicated; PA banding if congestive heart failure is due to large VSD; systemic–pulmonary shunt for severe PS
- Corrective Closure of VSD (total heart block common complication); relief of PS and/or valve replacement for significant tricuspid regurgitation; pacemaker implantation as indicated for complete heart block whether spontaneous or surgically induced.

Post-op: Regular follow-up is needed for possible progression of AV block and for routine pacemaker care if implanted. Limitation of activity is indicated if haemodynamic abnormalities exist.

Truncus arteriosus

Failure of normal septation and division of the common trunk into the pulmonary artery and aorta (Fig. 3.14).

Effect: A single vessel arises from both ventricles, straddling a VSD and providing blood flow to pulmonary, systemic and coronary circulation. Four types:

- Type 1 – main pulmonary artery arises from the truncus
- Type 2 – left and right pulmonary arteries arise separately from the back of the truncus
- Type 3 – left and right pulmonary arteries arise laterally from the truncus
- Type 4 – left and right pulmonary arteries arise laterally from the descending aorta.

Management:

- Palliative Pulmonary artery banding if excessive pulmonary flow, e.g. type 1. Systemic to pulmonary artery shunt to improve pulmonary flow if insufficient, e.g. type 4

Fig 3.14   Truncus arteriosus. A. Type 1. B. Type 2. C. Type 3. D. Type 4 (with permission from Park 2003)

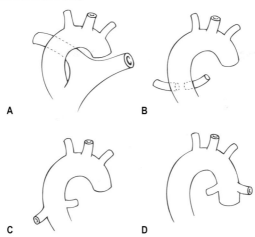

- Correction Usually within first few months: pulmonary arteries separated and conduit made from the right ventricle to the pulmonary circulation with closure of the VSD.

Post-op: Possibility of truncal valve regurgitation, ventricular arrhythmias.

Total anomalous pulmonary venous drainage (TAPVD)

Failure of the pulmonary veins to join the left atrium; instead, they are abnormally connected to the systemic venous circulation via the right atrium or veins draining towards it, e.g. SVC.

Four types, classified according to the pulmonary venous point of attachment:

- Supracardiac Most common – the common pulmonary vein drains into the SVC via the left SVC (vertical vein) and the left innominate vein (Fig. 3.15)
- Cardiac The common pulmonary vein drains into the coronary sinus or the pulmonary veins enter the right atrium separately through four openings
- Infracardiac (subdiaphragmatic) The common pulmonary vein drains into the portal vein, ductus venosus, hepatic vein or IVC
- Mixed type A combination of the other types.

Fig 3.15   Blood flow through the heart with supracardiac TAPVD (adapted with permission from Whaley & Wong 1991)

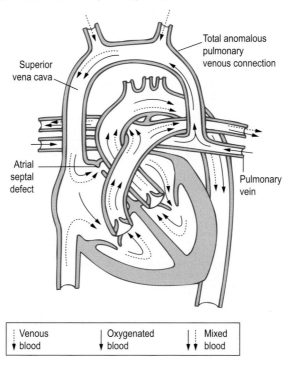

| ⋮ Venous | ↓ Oxygenated | ⋮⋮ Mixed |
| blood | blood | blood |

Effect: An interatrial communication is necessary for survival (PFO or ASD). If there is no obstruction to pulmonary venous return (most supracardiac and cardiac types), pulmonary venous return is large and there is only slight systemic arterial desaturation. If there is obstruction to pulmonary venous return (infracardiac type), pulmonary venous return is small and the infant is profoundly cyanosed.

Management: If obstructed, O_2, ventilation and diuretics to manage pulmonary oedema. ?Balloon septostomy to enlarge ASD. Surgical correction according to site of anomalous drainage – the aim is to channel pulmonary venous return to the left atrium, with closure of the ASD.

Post-op: Possibility of atrial arrhythmias.

Fig 3.16 Double-outflow right ventricle with (A) subaortic VSD, (B) subpulmonary VSD, (C) doubly committed VSD, (D) remote VSD (redrawn with permission from Royal Children's Hospital 2005)

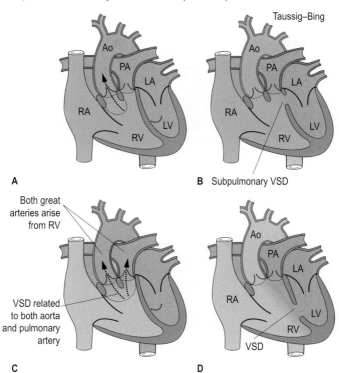

Double outlet right ventricle (DORV)

The aorta and pulmonary arteries arise side by side from the right ventricle (Fig. 3.16). The only outlet from the left ventricle is a large VSD. The aortic and pulmonary valves are at the same level. Subaortic and subpulmonary conuses separate the aortic and pulmonary valves from the tricuspid and mitral valves respectively. DORV may be subdivided according to the position of the VSD and further by the presence of pulmonary stenosis.

Effect:

- Subaortic VSD Oxygenated blood from the LV is directed to the aorta and desaturated systemic venous blood is directed to the PA

producing mild or no stenosis. In the absence of pulmonary stenosis the pulmonary blood flow is increased, resulting in congestive heart failure. The clinical picture resembles that of a large VSD with pulmonary hypertension and congestive heart failure

- Subpulmonary VSD Oxygenated blood from LV is directed to the PA and desaturated blood from the systemic vein is directed to the aorta, producing severe cyanosis. Pulmonary blood flow increases with the fall of the PVR. The clinical picture resembles TGA. Pulmonary vascular obstructive disease develops relatively early
- Doubly committed VSD In the presence of PS the clinical picture resembles that of Fallot's tetralogy. The large interventricular communication is located immediately beneath both the aortic and pulmonary valves
- Remote VSD The most complex type; the VSD is remote as it opens into the right ventricle beneath the tricuspid valve. Mild cyanosis is present and pulmonary blood flow is increased.

Management (adapted from Park 2003):

- Palliative
  - *Medical*: Treatment of congestive heart failure and SBE prophylaxis if indicated. For infants with large pulmonary blood flow and congestive heart failure – PA band
  - *Surgical*: For subpulmonary VSD, enlarge ASD by balloon or blade or atrial septectomy for increased mixing of pulmonary and systemic venous blood and decompression of the LA
  - For infants with PS and decreased pulmonary blood flow (Fallot type) S–P shunt if indicated.

- Corrective
  - *Subaortic VSD and doubly committed VSD:* creation of intraventricular tunnel between VSD and subaortic outflow tract by 6 months of age without PA banding
  - *Subpulmonary VSD:* intraventricular tunnel between the subpulmonary VSD and aorta is desirable. If not possible an intraventricular tunnel between VSD and PA (turns it into TGA) plus arterial switch operation during the first month of life, or Senning's operation (baffles to direct flow from SVC/IVC to RA and RV to PA; and from pulmonary veins to LA and LV to aorta)
  - *Fallot type:* intraventricular tunnel procedure (VSD to aorta) plus relief of PS by patch graft at 6 months–2 years of age or homograft valved conduit between RV and PA at 4–5 years
  - *Remote VSD:* when possible an intraventricular tunnel procedure (VSD to aorta) is preferred. If not possible, either a Fontan-type operation or Senning's operation plus closure of the VSD plus LV to aorta valved conduit placement is performed.

CONGENITAL HEART DEFECTS: SIGNS, SYMPTOMS AND DIAGNOSIS – AN OVERVIEW

Although each centre will have its own protocols, Table 3.1 may prove helpful in providing an overview of signs, symptoms and diagnostic pointers to assist initial recognition and management of congenital heart defects.

MYOCARDIAL DISEASE

Heart disease in childhood is not limited to anatomical arrangements and includes the following:

- Congenital Dilated, restrictive and obstructive cardiomyopathies have all been described as occurring congenitally. Endocardial fibroelastosis (which also occurs secondary to ventricular outflow tract obstruction) and hypertrophic obstructive cardiomyopathy are the two most common. Myocardial involvement can also occur in more systemic congenital disorders, e.g. hamartomas in tuberous sclerosis
- Infection Toxic cardiomyopathy is common in shock associated with septicaemia or toxic shock syndrome. The presentation of other infective illnesses such as rheumatic fever, botulism and typhoid may be predominantly via cardiac involvement. Viral myocarditis is not just a default diagnosis but has been traced to a variety of agents including Coxsackie, echo, rubella, herpes and influenza viruses (Pearson 2002).

HANDY HINTS FOR POST-OP MANAGEMENT

The goals of post-op cardiac management are to optimise cardiopulmonary support through external monitoring and to prevent secondary injury to the myocardium and other organs while providing effective analgesia/anxiolysis (Papo et al 1997).

Every centre that performs cardiac surgery will have its own guidelines for post-op care – the following are intended as general reminders:

1. Ascertain pre-op anatomy and type of surgery performed. If cardiopulmonary bypass was used, find out the duration of the bypass and cross-clamp time and whether there were any problems related to coming off bypass. Glean any other relevant information from surgical/anaesthetic staff – is there anything else they are concerned about that you need to be aware of?
2. Assessment to include:

A – Airway

- ET tube size and length
- Security of strapping
- Equal breath sounds on both sides of chest on auscultation.

Table 3.1 Signs, symptoms and diagnosis of congenital heart defects

Defect	Murmur	Heart failure	Cyanosis	Pulmonary blood flow	Blood pressure	Heart size	Chest X-ray	ECG	Comments/ presentation	Need Prostin
Coarctation	Systolic murmur radiating to back between scapula	Yes	No	Pulmonary venous congestion	Higher BP readings in arms	May be enlarged	Cardiomegaly, signs of pulmonary oedema, venous congestion	Baby RVH, older child may have LVH	Grey, collapsed, acidotic, no femoral pulses, hepatomegaly	Yes
Tetralogy of Fallot	Yes	No	Yes	Reduced	Normal	Normal	Boot shaped heart with concave MPA segment	RAD, RVH	Often ↑ Hb and haematocrit	Yes if very blue
Ventricular septal defect	Yes	Possibly	No	Increased	Usually normal	May be enlarged	Cardiomegaly, pulmonary oedema	Large VSD – LAH, LVH	Delayed growth and development, repeated pulmonary infection, CHF	No
Patent ductus arteriosus	Yes	Yes – if large duct	No	Increased pulmonary blood flow	Wide pulse pressure, low diastolic	May be enlarged if PDA large	If large PDA, cardiomegaly with LAE, LVE and increased PVM	CVH in large PDA, RVH if PVOD develops	If PDA large, CHF may develop	No
TGA	Yes if VSD, no if IVS	No	Yes – severe	Normal or minimally increased	Normal if VSD, lower with IVS	Narrow superior mediastinum	Egg-shaped heart	RAD, RVH	VSD present in 40% of cases	Yes
Truncus	Yes	Yes	mild	Increased pulmonary blood flow	Wide pulse pressure	Enlarged	Cardiomegaly, pulmonary oedema	CVH	Cyanosis often noted immediately after birth	No
Hypoplastic left heart syndrome	No	Yes	Yes	May have pulmonary venous congestion	Normal or low	Enlarged	Pulmonary vascular congestion if restrictive ASD	RVH and RAD	Mild cyanosis, tachycardia, tachypnoea, metabolic acidosis	Yes

				Pulmonary venous congestion			Pulmonary vascular congestion	RAD and RVH	Marked cyanosis and respiratory distress	Yes until echo
Obstructed total anomalous pulmonary venous drainage	No – but may have gallop rhythm	No	Severe		Normal or low	Normal or small because of decreased venous return to left heart				
PA	No	No	Severe	Reduced	Normal	Normal or enlarged	RA enlargement, MPA segment concave with decreased PVMs	Normal QRS axis, RAH	Severe and progressive cyanosis from birth	Yes
TA	Yes	No	Severe	Reduced	Normal	Normal or slightly enlarged	'Boot-shaped' heart with concave MPA segment	Superior QRS axis, RAH or CAH and LVH	Severe cyanosis, poor feeding, tachypnoea – 50% have VSD and PS – 20% have TGA	Yes
Critical AS	Yes – may be faint or absent in newborn	May develop	No	Normal or increased	Narrow pulse pressure	Normal or slightly enlarged	Usually normal	LVH	Weak, thready peripheral pulses	Yes
Ebstein's anomaly	Yes	Yes	Yes – most are cyanosed	Reduced	Normal	Extreme enlargement	Extreme cardiomegaly, particularly RA and decreased PVMS	RBBB, RAH WPW syndrome, SVT and AV block sometimes present	Cyanosis of newborns may improve as PVR falls – SVT is common	Yes

* NB In any presentation of a baby where a cardiac defect is suspected and the baby is cyanosed, Prostin should be started and then only discontinued on the advice of cardiologists or other specialists following echocardiogram

Abbreviations: ASD, atrial septal defect; AV, atrioventricular; CAH, combined atrial hypertrophy; CHF, congestive heart failure; CVH, common ventricular hypertrophy; IVS, intact ventricular septum; LAH, left atrial hypertrophy; LVH, left ventricular hypertrophy; MPA, main pulmonary artery; PDA, patent ductus arteriosus; PVM, pulmonary vascular marking; PVOD, pulmonary vascular obstructive disease; RA, right atrium; RAD, right axis deviation; RAH, right atrial hypertrophy; RBBB, right bundle branch block; RVH, right ventricular hypertrophy; SVT, supraventricular tachycardia; TGA, transposition of the great arteries; VSD, ventricular septal defect; WPW, Wolff–Parkinson–White.

Source: adapted from Heese 1992, Park 1997, Chang et al 1998 and Pearson 2002

B – Breathing

- Colour
- S_aO_2 – is this within an acceptable range given the procedure that has been performed? (Confirm S_aO_2 with blood co-oximetry measurement)
- Is nitric oxide (NO) being used?
- Chest movement, ventilation mode and settings
- Arterial blood gas analysis
- Chest X-ray will enable assessment of position of the ET tube, lung inflation, intravascular lines, drains and pacing wire placement.

C – Circulation

- Heart rate and rhythm
- BP/CVP/RAP/LAP/PAP and their wave forms; e.g. does the BP waveform look flat or 'damp'? Is this caused by poor cardiac output or a problem with the line itself?
- Drugs – is the child receiving infusions of inotropes/vasodilators? If so, check the dosage, rate and route and label lines clearly
- If drains are present, confirm position (chest X-ray), label and mark drainage on return from theatre. Most centres discard this total on fluid charts as drainage in theatre and calculate post-op losses only. 'Milk' cardiac chest drains initially and at 15 min–hourly intervals thereafter depending on drainage and local policy, to prevent blockage. Check drains are connected to thoracic suction at an appropriate pressure
- Are pacing wires in situ? If so, label (atrial/ventricular) and ensure that the metal ends are easily available should the child require pacing and that a pacing box is at the bedspace
- If the child is being paced, ascertain the underlying rate and rhythm and check with the surgeon/anaesthetist that the current settings on the pacing box are correct. A spare pacing box should be available
- Full set of bloods to include full blood count and clotting screen – may need treating
- Blood losses are usually replaced with whole blood or packed red cells
- Abnormal prothrombin or partial thromboplastin times are corrected with fresh frozen plasma (FFP) and by keeping platelet count within normal limits
- Low fibrinogen levels and other factor replacement can be corrected with cryoprecipitate
- If bleeding is above 10 ml/kg/h despite blood and replacement for coagulation deficiencies, surgical exploration may be required to assess location of bleeding.

Central nervous system

- Assess and record pupil size and reaction to light
- Administer analgesia as soon as child shows signs of waking from anaesthetic

- Consider giving bolus and then infusion – usually of opiates, e.g. morphine/fentanyl; monitor effect
- Muscle relaxants may be required to achieve synchrony with the ventilator (can also help to reduce the incidence of pulmonary hypertensive crisis).

Metabolic status

- Arterial blood gas analysis, mixed venous saturations and serum lactate to check the child is not hypoxaemic or hypercapnic and does not have a metabolic acidosis
- Blood taken for an electrolyte screen will enable any necessary corrections to be made and allow assessment of ionised calcium, blood sugar and magnesium levels.

Fluid management

- Maintenance fluids will be restricted (usually half to two-thirds maintenance), initially with added dextrose to prevent hypoglycaemia – check blood sugar level regularly
- Assess urine output – note and discard urine in catheter bag from theatre (as with chest drains); aim for 0.5–1 ml/kg/h initially
- To assess whether fluid management is effective:
  - Assess peripheral perfusion (pulses, capillary refill time)
  - Assess preload via central venous pressure (CVP), left atrial pressure (LAP) or both
  - Adequate urine output
  - Assess urea and electrolytes, Hb and haematocrit, urine specific gravity
  - Assess ongoing fluid losses through drains
  - Fluids are usually given in boluses of 5–10 ml/kg, monitoring preload and urine output
  - Nutritional support in the form of enteral or parenteral feeds is usually started within 48 hours of surgery.

CARDIOPULMONARY BYPASS

Cardiopulmonary bypass (CPB) is a mechanical means of circulating and oxygenating the patient's blood while diverting most of the circulation from the heart and lungs. During CPB the blood volume is circulated continuously between the patient and the bypass machine, where it is filtered, temperature-regulated and oxygenated.

The main factors involved in preventing complications of CPB are:

- Hypothermia Decreases tissue O_2 requirements, providing some protection against ischaemic injury
- Haemodilution The patient's blood is diluted with a crystalloid solution via the bypass machine to reduce blood viscosity and consequent formation of microthrombi
- Anticoagulation Heparinisation of blood to prevent coagulation in the bypass machine
- Cold cardioplegia Provides local hypothermia when infused into the aortic root and coronary arteries after aortic cross–clamping to induce cardiac standstill.

The risks of surgery involving CPB include:

- Infection
- Bleeding
- Microemboli, e.g. fat, air
- Platelet aggregation
- Cell haemolysis.

PROBLEMS

Cardiac tamponade

Cardiac tamponade after cardiac surgery is caused by fluid collecting within the pericardial sac, which impedes adequate diastolic relaxation and cardiac filling and impairs myocardial function. It occurs if mediastinal drainage is inadequate (hence the importance of meticulous management of chest drains) or if brisk bleeding related to poor coagulation occurs.

An acute manifestation of cardiac tamponade presents with a tachycardia, high CVP and LAP, and hypotension. Bradycardia is a late sign, which usually leads to cardiac arrest. Open pericardotomy is usually necessary to remove the fluid and therefore the pressure within the pericardium.

Pulmonary hypertensive crisis

Pulmonary hypertensive crisis is characterised by an acute rise in PA pressure followed by a reduction in cardiac output and a fall in arterial O_2 saturation. It occurs more commonly with certain cardiac defects, e.g. TGA, VSD, AVSD, truncus arteriosus. Management includes prophylaxis in those at risk by avoiding factors that lead to increased pulmonary vascular resistance, e.g. acidosis (P_{CO_2} pH – aim for normal P_{CO_2} or mild alkalosis), pain (ensure effective analgesia and sedation is administered). NO may be used to improve pulmonary vasodilatation.

In the event of a pulmonary hypertensive crisis, treatment includes rapid hand bagging with 100% O_2 and boluses of IV sedation, e.g. morphine/fentanyl, together with muscle relaxants.

CARDIAC OUTPUT

Cardiac output is the amount of blood ejected by each ventricle (in litres or millilitres) per minute. Normal cardiac output is higher per kilogram of body weight in the child than in the adult.

- 400 ml/kg/min at birth
- 200 ml/kg/min within first weeks of life
- 100 ml/kg/min during adolescence (Hazinski 1992).

$$\text{Cardiac output} = \text{Stroke volume} \times \text{Heart rate}$$

$$\text{Preload} = \text{Afterload} \times \text{Contractility.}$$

In order to obtain the 'normal' cardiac output for children of different ages and sizes, the cardiac index is calculated.

$$\text{Cardiac index} = \frac{\text{Cardiac output}}{\text{Body surface area (m}^2\text{)}}$$

Normal range $= 3.5$–$5.5 \ l/min/m^2$ body surface area (Shemie 1997).

Cardiac output is a prime determinant of haemodynamic function and in the critically ill child should be evaluated as either adequate or inadequate to meet the child's metabolic demands.

Preload is the amount of myocardial fibre stretch that is present before contraction and is related to the volume of blood in the ventricles prior to contraction, CVP and LAP (Starling's law). Frank Starling's law observed that normal myocardium generates greater tension during contraction if it is stretched before contraction. However, fibre length is not readily measured and therefore preload or ventricular end-diastolic pressure is monitored as an indirect measurement.

Factors affecting preload: ventricular compliance, tachycardia.

Afterload refers to the resistance to ejection from a ventricle. Ventricular afterload is the sum of all forces opposing ventricular emptying. A decrease in afterload is often associated with an improvement in ventricular function. Because fibre shortening occurs only when the ventricle has generated sufficient tension to equal its afterload, an increase in ventricular afterload reduces contraction time and thus the stroke volume of the ventricle. It is also related to Poiseuille's law, which states that pressure is a product of flow and resistance:

$$\text{Pressure} = \text{Flow} \times \text{Resistance}$$

From this equation, an increase in resistance will be associated with a decrease in flow (stroke volume) unless pressure increases. Even a normal afterload may be excessive when myocardial function is poor.

Contractility refers to the strength and efficiency of contraction; it is the force generated by the myocardium, independent of preload and afterload. Contractility is reduced by many factors, including hypoxia, acidosis, excessive preload/afterload, hypocalcaemia and nutritional deficiencies.

INVASIVE INTRAVASCULAR PRESSURE MONITORING

Following cardiac surgery various lines will be in situ in order to continuously monitor the child's cardiovascular status.

Fig 3.17 Arterial waveform (redrawn with permission from C&S Solutions 2006, www.cssolutions.biz)

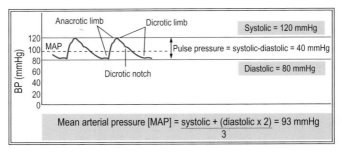

Fig 3.18 Central venous pressure waveform. This is created by the pressure changes occurring in the right atrium during right atrial systole and diastole and consists of the A wave, C wave, X descent, V and Y descent as shown here. The A wave is generated during atrial systole and its height is a direct result of how much pressure is occurring in the atrium as the blood is being ejected into the ventricle (redrawn with permission from C&S Solutions 2006, www.cssolutions.biz)

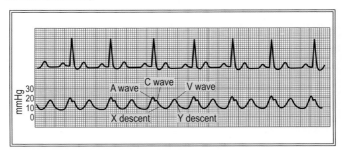

Intra-arterial pressure

Intra-arterial pressure monitoring is the only way to continuously measure the child's blood pressure. The systolic (higher) figure is the pressure when the ventricles contract and the diastolic (lower) figure is the pressure when the ventricles are relaxing and filling. The normal arterial pulse contour has a sharp upstroke during rapid ejection, followed by slow ejection and subsequent decrease (see Fig. 3.17). The dicrotic notch denotes the end of ejection and closure of the aortic valve. Estimates can be made of cardiac output based on the quality of the arterial pulse contour. Low cardiac output may show a narrowing pulse pressure.

Atrial pressure

Atrial pressure is an indirect measurement of ventricular preload. It should be remembered that interpretation of the measurements depends on the compliance of the ventricle and normal functioning of the AV valve.

- Right atrial (RA) pressure Directly measured via RA line inserted during surgery; indirectly measured via CVP line (see Fig. 3.18)
- Left atrial (LA) pressure Directly measured via LA line inserted at time of surgery; indirectly measured via pulmonary capillary wedge pressure, achieved through inflation of balloon tip of Swan–Ganz catheter.

Pulmonary artery catheterisation (Swan–Ganz)

A balloon-tipped, flow-directed catheter is inserted into the pulmonary artery (see Fig. 3.19) to allow measurement of cardiac output (equipped with a thermistor) and right atrial, pulmonary arterial and pulmonary capillary wedge pressures, together with mixed venous saturations (Table 3.2).

Table 3.2 Information derived from pulmonary artery catheterisation	
Variable	**Normal range**
Haemodynamic	
Stroke index	30–60 ml/m^2
Cardiac index	3.5–5.5 l/min/m^2
O$_2$ transport	
Arterial O$_2$ content	17–20 ml/dl
Mixed venous content	12–15 ml/dl
O$_2$ availability	550–650 ml/min/m^2
O$_2$ consumption	120–200 ml/min/m^2

Souce: adapted from Shemie 1997.

Fig 3.19   Pulmonary artery catheter insertion and flotation (redrawn with permission from C&S Solutions 2006, www.cssolutions.biz)

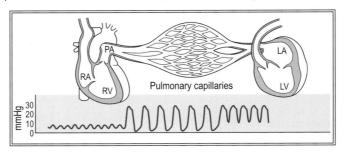

Pulmonary arterial diastolic pressure may accurately reflect left atrial pressure only when the pulmonary vascular resistance is normal.

THE NORMAL ELECTROCARDIOGRAM (ECG)

An ECG measures the electrical activity of the heart and records it on graph paper. This allows the sequence and magnitude of the electrical impulses generated by the heart to be analysed and evaluated (Fig. 3.20).

Information supplied by the ECG includes:

• Heart rate and rhythm
• Abnormalities of conduction
• Muscular damage (ischaemia)
• Hypertrophy
• Effects of electrolyte imbalance
• Influence of various drugs
• Pericardial disease.

The contraction of any muscle is associated with electrical changes called depolarisation, and these changes can be detected by electrodes attached to the surface of the body. Although the heart has four chambers, from the electrical point of view it can be thought of as having only two, as the atria contract together and then the ventricles contract together.

The electrical discharge for each cycle starts in the sinoatrial (SA) node in the right atrium. Depolarisation then spreads through the atrial muscle fibres. There is a delay while depolarisation spreads through the atrioventricular (AV) node (also in the right atrium). The conduction is then very rapid down specialised conduction tissue – first a single pathway, the 'bundle of His', then this divides in the septum between the ventricles into right and left bundle branches. The left bundle branch divides itself into two. Conduction spreads rapidly through the mass of the ventricular

Fig 3.20   A. Normal ECG trace (sinus rhythm). B. Labelled portion of sinus rhythm

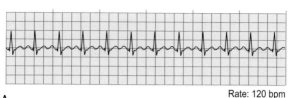

A   Rate: 120 bpm

B

muscle through specialised tissue called 'Purkinje fibres'. Repolarisation then takes place – the return of the ventricular mass to the electrical state (Hampton 1992).

- The P wave represents the contraction and depolarisation of the atria. Their muscle mass is relatively small and the electrical charge accompanying their contraction is therefore also small
- The PR interval represents the time taken for the impulse to spread from the SA node, through the atrial muscle and the AV node, down the bundle of His and into the ventricular muscle
- The QRS complex represents ventricular depolarisation. As the ventricles are large, there is a large deflection of the ECG when they contract
- The T wave represents the return of the ventricular mass to the resting electrical state (repolarisation).

ARRHYTHMIAS

Arrhythmias are deviations from the normal (sinus) rhythm of the heart. Arrhythmias that require immediate treatment in the child are those that significantly decrease cardiac output or systemic perfusion.

There are three main classifications:

- Bradyarrhythmias Too slow for the child's clinical condition
- Tachyarrhythmias Too fast for the child's clinical condition
- Collapse rhythms Ineffective conduction that is unable to sustain cardiac output.

Examples of bradyarrhythmias

Sinus bradycardia (Fig. 3.21)

Characteristics of sinus rhythm are present. Heart rate below 80 beats per minute (bpm) in newborn infants and below 60 bpm in older children may be significant.

Causes: Vagal stimulation, hypoxia, hypotension, raised intracranial pressure, hypothermia, hyperkalaemia, beta-blocking drugs.

Treatment: Treat underlying cause promptly.

Junctional (nodal) rhythm (Fig. 3.22)

The P wave may be absent or QRS complexes are followed by inverted P waves. If there is persistent failure of the SA node, the AV node may act as the main pacemaker, with a relatively slow rate (40–60 bpm).

Causes: May occur in otherwise normal heart after cardiac surgery, digitalis toxicity, in conditions with increased vagal tone, e.g. raised intracranial pressure.

Significance: Slow heart rate may significantly decrease cardiac output and produce symptoms.

Treatment: No treatment is indicated if the child is asymptomatic. Treatment is directed to digitalis toxicity if this is the cause.

Fig 3.21   Sinus bradycardia

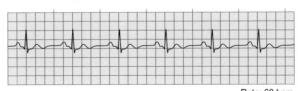

Rate: 60 bpm

Fig 3.22   Junctional (nodal) rhythm

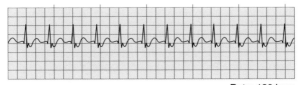

Rate: 120 bpm

Heart (AV) block

This is a disturbance in conduction between the normal sinus impulse and the eventual ventricular response. It is classified according to the severity of the conduction disturbance.

First-degree heart block (Fig. 3.23)

Abnormally prolonged PR interval due to a delay in conduction through the AV node.

Cause: Present in some healthy children, cardiomyopathies, congenital heart defects, e.g. ASD, Ebstein's anomaly, following cardiac surgery, digitalis toxicity.

Significance: Usually no treatment indicated except in digitalis toxicity.

Second-degree heart block (Fig. 3.24)

Some but not all P waves are followed by QRS complexes (dropped beats). There are several types:

Mobitz type I (Wenckebach phenomenon)

The PR interval becomes progressively prolonged until one QRS complex is dropped completely.

Fig 3.23 First degree heart block

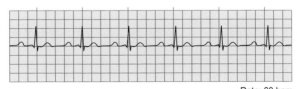

Rate: 60 bpm

Fig. 3.24 Second degree heart block Mobitz type 1 (Wenckebach phenomenon) (with permission from Park 1997)

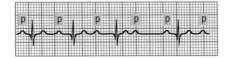

Cause: Myocarditis, cardiomyopathy, myocardial infarction, congenital heart disease, cardiac surgery, digitalis toxicity; also affects otherwise healthy children.

Significance: The block is at the level of the AV node. Usually does not progress to complete heart block.

Treatment: Treat underlying cause.

Mobitz Type II (Fig. 3.25)

The AV conduction is all or none; there is either normal AV conduction or the conduction is completely blocked.

Cause: As for Mobitz type I.

Significance: The block is at the level of the bundle of His. It is more serious than type I block, since it may progress to complete heart block.

Treatment: Treat underlying cause. Prophylactic pacemaker therapy may be indicated.

Two-to-one (or higher) AV block (Fig. 3.26)

A QRS complex follows every second (third or fourth) P wave, resulting in 2:1 (3:1 or 4:1 respectively) AV block.

Cause: Similar to other second degree AV blocks.

Fig 3.25 Second degree heart block Mobitz type II (with permission from Park 2003)

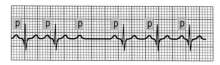

Fig 3.26 2:1 (higher) heart block (with permission from Park 2003)

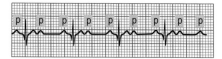

Significance: The block is usually at the AV nodal level and occasionally at the level of the bundle of His. It may occasionally progress to complete heart block.

Treatment: The underlying cause is treated. Electrophysiological studies may be necessary to determine the level of the block. Occasional pacemaker therapy.

Third-degree or complete heart block (Fig. 3.27)

Atrial and ventricular activities are entirely independent of one another. P waves and P–P intervals are regular at a heart rate reasonable for the child's age. QRS complexes are also regular but at a much slower rate than the P rate.

Causes: Maternal lupus erythematosus; congenital type may be isolated or associated with congenital heart disease, e.g. TGA. Acquired type is usually a complication of cardiac surgery. Rarely, severe myocarditis, mumps, diphtheria, tumours in the conduction system, overdose of certain drugs. May follow myocardial infarction. These causes produce either temporary or permanent heart block.

Significance: Congestive heart failure may develop in infancy, particularly if congenital heart defect is present. Children with isolated complete heart block can be asymptomatic in childhood.

Treatment: No treatment is indicated for asymptomatic congenital complete heart block. Temporary ventricular pacemaker is indicated for children with transient heart block. Permanent artificial ventricular pacemaker is indicated for children with surgically induced heart block and those who are asymptomatic or have congestive heart failure (Park 2003).

Consider:
- If increased vagal tone or primary AV block give atropine:
  - First dose 0.02 mg/kg – may repeat
  - Minimum dose 0.1 mg
  - Maximum dose for child 1 mg
- Cardiac pacing

Fig 3.27 Third-degree or complete heart block (with permission from Park 2003)

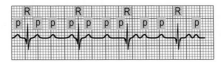

Examples of tachyarrhythmias

Sinus tachycardia (Fig. 3.28)

The characteristics of sinus rhythm are present. A rate above 140 bpm in children and above 160 bpm in infants may be significant. The heart rate is usually lower than 200 bpm.

Causes: Pain, anxiety, fever, hypovolaemia, circulatory shock, anaemia, congestive heart failure, myocardial disease.

Significance: Increased cardiac work is well tolerated by the healthy myocardium.

Treatment: Treat the underlying cause. Refer to Figure 3.22.

Supraventricular tachycardia (Fig. 3.29)

SVT in infants generally produces a heart rate of more than 220 bpm, and often 250–300 bpm. Lower rates occur in children during SVT. The QRS complex is narrow, making differentiation between marked sinus tachycardia due to shock and SVT difficult, particularly because SVT may also be associated with poor systemic perfusion.

Fig 3.28 Sinus tachycardia

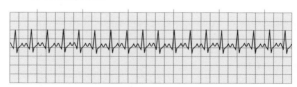

Rate: 170 bpm

Fig 3.29 Supraventricular tachycardia (SVT)

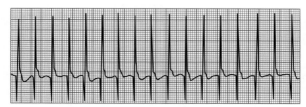

The following characteristics may help to distinguish between sinus tachycardia and SVT:

- Sinus tachycardia is typically characterised by a heart rate less than 200 bpm in infants and children whereas infants with SVT typically have a heart rate greater than 200 bpm
- P waves may be difficult to identify in both sinus tachycardia and SVT once the ventricular rate exceeds 200 bpm. If P waves are identifiable, they are usually upright in leads I and AVF in sinus tachycardia while they are negative in leads II, III and AVF in SVT
- In sinus tachycardia, the heart rate varies from beat to beat and is often unresponsive to stimulation, but there is no beat-to-beat variability in SVT
- Termination of SVT is abrupt whereas the heart rate slows gradually in sinus tachycardia in response to treatment
- A history consistent with shock (e.g. gastroenteritis or septicaemia) is usually present with sinus tachycardia (Advanced Life Support Group 2006).

Causes: No demonstrable heart disease present in many children. Some congenital cardiac defects, e.g. Ebstein's anomaly, TGA, are more prone to this arrhythmia.

Table 3.3 Guidelines for the drug treatment of tachycardia

The following are only guidelines as to the initial treatment of a specific arrhythmia; expert advice should be sought before prescribing or if there is a lack of response.

Arrhythmia	Initial treatment
Supraventricular tachycardia	1. Adenosine – repeat bolus when necessary 2. Digoxin 3. Propranolol 4. Flecainide 5. Verapamil
Sinus tachycardia Atrial fibrillation Atrial flutter Atrial tachycardia	Find and treat underlying cause 1. Digoxin 2. Propranolol 3. Amiodarone
Ventricular tachycardia	1. Amiodarone 2. Lignocaine (if no access or only drug available) 3. Magnesium sulphate
Wolff–Parkinson–White syndrome with atrial fibrillation	1. Amiodarone **Do not give digoxin or verapamil**

Source: reproduced with permission from Guy's, St. Thomas', King's College and University Lewisham Hospitals 2005.

Fig 3.30 Algorithm for the management of supraventricular tachycardia (with permission from Advanced Life Support Group 2005)

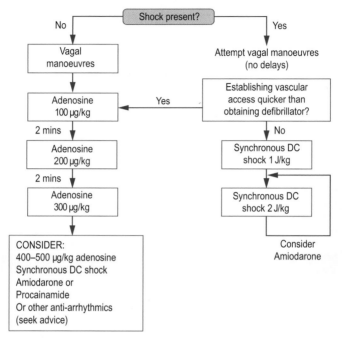

Vagal manoeuvres

These include:

- Application of rubber glove filled with iced water over face – or wrapping infant in towel and immersing face in iced water for 5 seconds
- One-sided carotid sinus massage
- Valsalva manoeuvre, e.g. blowing hard through a straw
- **Do not use ocular pressure in infants or children** as may cause damage.

Significance: It may decrease cardiac output and result in congestive cardiac failure – if this develops the infant's/child's condition can deteriorate rapidly. Cardiopulmonary stability during episodes of SVT is affected by the child's age, duration of SVT and prior ventricular function and

Fig 3.31   Junctional ectopic tachycardia (with permission from Legras 1997)

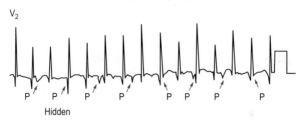

ventricular rate. If baseline myocardial function is impaired, SVT can produce signs of shock in a relatively short time.

Junctional ectopic tachycardia (JET; Fig. 3.31)

Narrow QRS complex tachycardia with a rate of more than 120 bpm in the presence of AV dissociation; in this case, the ventricular rate is faster than the atrial rate.

Causes: Most frequent in patients with pre-op and residual right ventricular hypertension. Extensive surgery near the AV node with structural or hypoxic damage is an important factor, as are post-op pyrexia and high levels of circulating catecholamines.

Significance: Considered one of the most refractory and lethal of the post-op arrhythmias – does not respond to cardioversion, difficult to treat medically, results in the loss of AV synchrony in patients immediately after complex cardiac surgery.

Treatment:

- Treat hypovolaemia and fever
- Correct hypokalaemia to 4–5 mmol/l within 1–2 h
- Patient should be sedated, paralysed and cooled to 35°C core prior to the use of drugs
- Inotropes should be reduced as much as possible
- Once tachycardia reduces to less than 160 bpm, atrial pacing at approximately 10 bpm faster than JET may provide AV synchrony and suppress this arrhythmia
- Antiarrhythmic drugs, e.g. amiodarone, may be indicated if no response is achieved by the above management
- If all other treatment fails, extracorporeal membrane oxygenation (ECMO) may be useful because JET tends to resolve over time (Legras 1997).

Fig 3.32 Atrial fibrillation

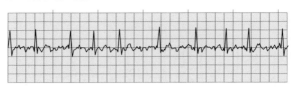

Rate: 100 bpm

Atrial fibrillation (Fig. 3.32)

Atrial fibrillation is characterised by an extremely fast atrial rate (flutter wave at 350–600 bpm) and an irregular ventricular response with normal QRS complexes.

Causes: Structural heart disease with dilated atria, myocarditis, previous surgery involving atria, digitalis toxicity.

Significance: Rapid ventricular rate and the loss of coordinated contraction of the atria and the ventricles decrease cardiac output. Atrial thrombus formation may occur.

Treatment: Digoxin is given to slow the ventricular rate and propranolol may be added if necessary. Cardioversion may be indicated, but recurrence is common. Patients should preferably be anticoagulated for 3–4 weeks before and after cardioversion to prevent embolisation of atrial thrombus.

Wolff–Parkinson–White (WPW) syndrome (Fig. 3.33)

WPW syndrome is characterised by a short PR interval, and the QRS complex shows an early slurred upstroke called a delta wave.

Significance: Results from an anomalous conduction pathway between the atrium and the ventricle, bypassing the normal delay of conduction in the AV node. Children with WPW syndrome are prone to sustained attacks of SVT (Park 1997).

Fig 3.33 Wolff–Parkinson–White syndrome

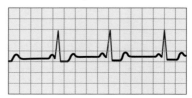

Pacing

Arrhythmias may be exacerbated by electrolyte disturbances. Most are short-lived and asymptomatic. When treatment is required a preference for pacing solutions reflects:

- the opportunity provided by the pacing wires
- the preponderance of bradycardias, usually due to varying degrees of AV dissociation
- the negative inotropic effects of antiarrhythmic drugs.

Therapeutic cooling can also be used for drug- and pacing-resistant tachyarrhythmias (e.g. JET) if evidence suggests they are significantly affecting cardiac output. Elective hypothermia requires mandatory paralysis.

Convention dictates that perioperative epicardial pacing wires are positioned with atrial wires to the right chest and ventricular wires to the left. Without this access, short-term solutions for bradyarrhythmias may be achieved with transcutaneous or transoesophageal pacing while a transvenous wire is positioned.

The most frequent indication for pacing is bradyarrhythmia. In children the fall in output with bradycardia is precipitate and dramatic. Even in older children and adults the ability to abruptly compensate by increasing stroke volume is limited. The indication for pacing a brady-arrhythmia is clinical evidence of a low cardiac output: altered conscious level, syncope, low urine output, poor peripheral perfusion, acidosis or hypotension (Pearson 2002).

There are three basic concepts associated with pacing:

- Capturing Whether the pacemaker is pacing the desired chamber(s)
- Sensing Whether the pacemaker is sensing the patient's own (intrinsic) contractions of the heart chambers. This is necessary so that the pacemaker avoids competition with the patient's own rhythm. The pacemaker only 'kicks in' when it cannot detect (sense) the patient's own effort
- Threshold The least amount of stimulus required to stimulate the myocardium or the least amount of voltage for the patient's own beats to be sensed (Horrocks 2002).

Pacing modes are described by a standard terminology that describes in sequence the chambers: paced, sensed and the mode of pacing (Tables 3.4 and 3.5).

It is important for appropriately trained and skilled medical staff to undertake pacemaker checks once/twice daily. There should be spare pacemakers available in case of failure/problems – some units may use a variety of models.

Table 3.4	Pacemaker terminology			
Chamber paced	**Chamber sensed**	**Response to sensing**	**Programmability**	**Tachyarrhythmia functions**
0 = None	0 = None	0 = None	0 = None	0 = None
A = Atrium	A = Atrium	T = Triggered	P = Programme	P = Pace (overdrive)
V = Ventricle	V = Ventricle	I = Inhibited	M = Multiprogramme	S = Shock
D = Dual	D = Dual	D = Dual (T + I)	R = Rate modulation	D = Dual P + S

Source: adapted from Pearson 2002

Table 3.5	Mapping pacing terminology
Fixed rate pacing	A00 or V00
Atrial demand pacing	AAI
Ventricular demand pacing	VVI
AV sequential pacing	DVI
AV universal	DDD
AV demand	DDI

Source: adapted from Pearson 2002

Examples of collapse rhythms

It is assumed that basic life support measures to assess and maintain:

- Airway
- Breathing and
- Circulation

have been initiated.

Ventricular fibrillation (VF)

VF is characterised by bizarre complexes at varying sizes and configuration. The rate is rapid and irregular. See Fig. 3.35.

Causes: Post-op state, severe hypoxia, hyperkalaemia, digitalis, myocardial infarction, some drugs (e.g. anaesthetics).

Significance: Can be fatal, since it results in ineffective circulation.

Treatment: Refer to Figure 3.34.

Fig. 3.34   Paediatric advanced life support (with permission from
Resuscitation Council (UK) 2005)

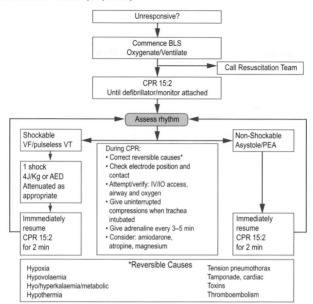

Fig 3.35   Ventricular fibrillation

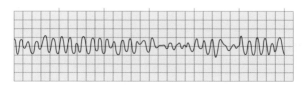

Ventricular tachycardia (VT; Fig. 3.36)

VT is characterised by rapid, wide QRS complexes (rate of 120–200 bpm)
with an absence of P waves. The QRS complexes are slightly irregular
and vary slightly in shape.

Causes: Cardiomyopathy, cardiac tumours, pre- or post-op, congenital
heart disease, digitalis toxicity, certain drugs including antibiotics, antihistamines, insecticides and some anaesthetic agents.

Fig 3.36   Ventricular tachycardia

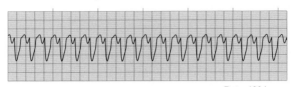

Rate: 180 bpm

Fig 3.37   Algorithm for the management of ventricular tachycardia (with permission from Advanced Life Support Group 2006)

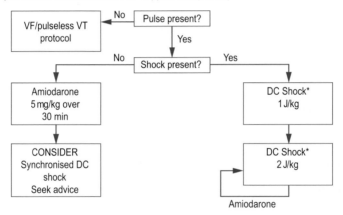

Significance: Usually signifies a serious myocardial pathology or dysfunction. Cardiac output may decrease notably and deteriorate to VF.

Treatment: Check whether pulse is present. If not, refer to algorithm in Figure 3.34. If pulse is present, synchronised cardioversion is required at 1 J/kg. See Fig 3. 37.

Consider following text for further clarification.

Early treatment of ventricular tachycardia (with pulse) (Advanced Life Support Group 2006)

- Early consultation with paediatric cardiologist
- May suggest use of amiodarone or procainamide – both can cause hypotension, which should be treated with volume expansion.

Fig 3.38   Asystole

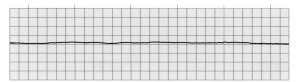

- Where VT has been caused by drug toxicity, sedation, anaesthesia and DC shock may be the safest approach – use synchronised shocks initially as these are less likely to produce VF but, if they are ineffectual, subsequent attempts will have to be asynchronous if the child is in shock
- The treatment of torsades de pointes VT is magnesium sulphate by IV infusion (25–50 mg/kg (max 2 g)
- Amiodarone 5 mg/kg may be given over a few minutes in VT if the child is in severe shock
- Seek advice.

Asystole (Fig. 3.38)

Asystole is characterised by a straight line on the ECG monitor, with P waves occasionally observed.

Causes: Respiratory arrest, myocardial infarction.

Significance: Diagnosed by the absence of a palpable central pulse accompanied by apnoea, together with absent cardiac electrical activity.

Treatment: Refer to PALS algorithm in Figure 3.34.

Pulseless electrical activity (PEA)

This was previously known as electromechanical dissociation or EMD. There are recognised complexes seen on the ECG monitor but there is an absence of palpable pulses and inadequate cardiac output.

Causes: Include four Hs and four Ts:

- Hypovolaemia (most common cause)
- Hypothermia
- Hypoxaemia
- Hyperkalaemia
- Tamponade
- Tension pneumothorax

- Thromboembolism
- Toxicity – i.e. drug overdose (commonly tricyclic antidepressant).

Significance: The underlying cause of PEA must be sought but PEA should be treated and managed like asystole until the specific cause has been identified and treated.

Treatment: See PALS algorithm in Figure 3.34.

REFERENCES

Advanced Life Support Group 2006 Available on line at www.alsg.org
C&S Solutions 2006 Hemodynamic monitoring Part I: Waveform recognition. Screen shots. C&S Solutions, Vincennes, IN. Available on line at: www.cssolutions.biz/hemo1s.html
Cincinnati Childrens Hospital Medical Center 2004 Interrupted aortic arch/ventricular septal defect. Cincinnati Childrens Hospital Medical Center, Cincinnati, OH. Available on line at www.cincinattichildrens.org/health/heart-encyclopaedia/anomalies/iaa.htm
Guy's, St. Thomas', King's College and University Lewisham Hospitals 2005 Paediatric formulary, 7th edn. Guy's, St Thomas' and Lewisham Hospitals, London
Hampton JR 1992 The ECG made easy, 4th edn. Churchill Livingstone, Edinburgh
Hazinski MF (ed) 1992 Nursing care of the critically ill child, 2nd edn. CV Mosby, St. Louis, MO
Heese HdeV 1992 Handbook of paediatrics, 4th edn. Oxford University Press, Cape Town
Horrocks F 2002 Manual of neonatal and paediatric heart disease. Whurr, London
Jonas RA 2003 Congenital heart disease: update on the Norwood procedure for hypoplastic left heart syndrome. Heart Views 4(3). Available on line at: www.hmc.org.qa/hmc/heartviews/H-V-v4%20N3/5.htm
Legras MD 1997 Arrhythmias in the pediatric intensive care unit. In: Singh NL (ed) Manual of pediatric critical care. WB Saunders, Philadelphia, PA
Papo MC, Hernan LJ, Fuhrman BP 1997 Postoperative cardiac care for congenital heart disease. In: Singh NL (ed) Manual of pediatric critical care. WB Saunders, Philadelphia, PA
Park MK 1997 The pediatric cardiology handbook, 2nd edn. CV Mosby, St. Louis, MO
Park MK 2003 The pediatric cardiology handbook, 3rd edn. CV Mosby, St Louis, MO
Pearson G 2002 Handbook of paediatric intensive care. WB Saunders, Edinburgh

Resuscitation Council (UK) 2005 Resuscitation guidelines.
Resuscitation Council (UK), London. Available on line at:
www.resus.org.uk

Royal Children's Hospital 2005 Double outlet right ventricle. Royal
Children's Hospital, London. Available on line at: www.rch.org.au/
cardiology/defects

Sano S, Ishino K, Kawada M et al 2003 Right ventricle–pulmonary artery
shunt in first-stage palliation of hypoplastic left heart syndrome.
J Thorac Cardiovasc Surg 126: 504–509

Shemie SD 1997 Cardiovascular monitoring. In: Singh N L (ed) Manual
of pediatric critical care. WB Saunders, Philadelphia, PA

Whaley LF, Wong DL 1991 Nursing care of infants and children, 4th edn.
CV Mosby, St Louis, MO

Williams C, Asquith J (eds) 2000 Paediatric intensive care nursing.
Churchill Livingstone, Edinburgh

Wilson KJW 1987 Ross and Wilson anatomy and physiology in health and
illness, 6th edn. Churchill Livingstone, Edinburgh

FURTHER READING

Bacha EA, Daves S, Hardin J et al 2006 Single-ventricle palliation for
high-risk neonates: the emergence of an alternative hybrid stage I
strategy. J Thor Cardiovasc Surg 131: 163–171

RENAL DYSFUNCTION

4

Renal failure is the inability of the kidneys to excrete waste products, concentrate urine, regulate electrolyte concentration and maintain pH.

Acute renal failure is the sudden loss or deterioration of kidney function with a progressive rise of serum creatinine and urea. Other characteristics include disturbance in fluid balance, acid–base balance and hyperkalaemia.

Box 4.1   Normal values

Urea	2.5–7.5 mmol/l
Creatinine	40–90 µmol/l
Potassium	3.5–5 mmol/l
Sodium	135–145 mmol/l

ACUTE RENAL FAILURE

Acute renal failure (ARF) is the sudden loss or deterioration of kidney function with a progressive rise of serum creatinine and urea. This may be accompanied by oliguria (<1 ml/kg/h) or occasionally polyuria. Other characteristics include a disturbance in fluid balance, acid–base balance and hyperkalaemia. The causes of ARF are commonly classified according to the location of the primary disorder:

1. **Prerenal** Disordered perfusion of a kidney that is structurally normal. Situations causing reduced blood flow to the kidney include:
   - Poor myocardial function
   - Cardiac surgery
   - Reduced blood volume, e.g. trauma
   - Moderate to severe dehydration
   - Septic shock, e.g. meningococcaemia

   Correcting the underperfusion may correct the renal failure.
2. **Intrinsic** Damage to kidney function: glomerulus/tubules/renal vasculature. Causes include:
   - Uncorrected prerenal ARF, e.g. persistent shock with meningococcaemia
   - Drug toxicity, e.g. gentamicin

- Primary renal disease, e.g. haemolytic uraemic syndrome.
Non-reversible – fluid resuscitation will not improve urine output.
3. **Postrenal** Disordered urinary drainage: refers to any obstructive lesion beyond the renal tubule. Causes include:
  - Involvement of postureteral valves
  - Congenital abnormality
  - Related to blood clots, calculi, tumours
  - Trauma.
  Treatment requires accurate assessment of the cause; if this can be corrected swiftly, intrinsic renal failure may be avoided.

Methods of treating acute renal failure in the critically ill child are:

- Peritoneal dialysis (PD)
- Continuous veno-venous haemofiltration (CVVH)
- Continuous veno-venous haemodiafiltration (CVVHD)
- Haemodialysis.

See Table 4.1 for the advantages and disadvantages of types of treatment.

PROCESSES INVOLVED IN FLUID AND SOLUTE REMOVAL

- Solute removal by **diffusion** – the movement of solutes down their concentration gradients, from regions of higher to lower concentration, until uniformity is reached
- Movement of water by **ultrafiltration** – the movement of fluid (water) down a pressure gradient, i.e. from a region of high pressure on one side of the membrane to a region of low pressure on the other

Table 4.1 Advantages and disadvantages of various modalities of renal replacement therapy for acute renal failure

Type	Complexity	Use in hypotension	Efficiency	Volume control	Anti-coagulation
Peritoneal dialysis	Low	Yes	Moderate	Moderate	No
Intermittent dialysis	Moderate	No	High	Moderate	Yes
Continuous veno-venous haemofiltration	Moderate	Yes	Moderate	Good	Yes
Continuous veno-venous haemodiafiltration	High	Yes	High	Good	Yes

Source: with permission from Strazdins et al 2004.

- Removal of solutes by **convection** – the movement of solutes with a water flow (solvent drag), e.g. the movement of membrane-permeable solutes with ultrafiltered water. Although the convection associated with ultrafiltration results in some solute transfer, this is primarily by passive diffusion
- Movement of water by **osmosis** – the movement of water through a membrane from an area of high to low water concentration. During osmosis water molecules move across the membrane to the side containing a higher concentration of osmotically active particles.

PERITONEAL DIALYSIS (PD)

PD has generally been the preferred method of managing the critically ill child in acute renal failure but may be contraindicated by an acute surgical abdomen or access difficulties, diaphragmatic splinting causing problems with mechanical ventilation, and catheter malfunction.

PD involves the introduction of dialysis fluid into the peritoneal cavity through a catheter placed in the lower part of the abdomen. The peritoneum serves as the dialysis membrane. This is intracorporeal blood purification as no blood ever leaves the body of the patient.

An osmotic pressure gradient is applied by the addition to the dialysis fluid of an osmotic agent, glucose, which draws water from the blood. The concentration of glucose is chosen according to the fluid removal required.

Solutes are transported across the membrane by diffusion, the concentration gradient being between the blood and the PD fluid. Waste products present in the blood perfusing the peritoneum will diffuse from the blood vessels into the dialysis fluid.

When the dialysis fluid is drained from the abdominal cavity, it contains waste products and excess fluid extracted from the blood.

Fluid and solute removal in PD is controlled by:

- glucose concentration
- dwell time
- volume
- peritoneal membrane characteristics.

Some solutes are transported from the PD fluid to the blood during dialysis – hence the PD fluid needs to contain sufficient amounts of a buffer source particularly important during bicarbonate PD.

Bags of fluid for bicarbonate PD in the acidotic patient are made up in pharmacy in most centres and can be ordered as required.

The following details need to be prescribed

1. **Exchange volume** 20–30 ml/kg is generally effective. It will take a longer time for the concentration gradient to decline in a large volume of fluid. In the critically ill child, it may be necessary to use the smaller volume because of cardiovascular instability. PD can also be of value when used for cooling purposes in the critically ill child with a pyrexia that is unresponsive to other antipyretic therapy. In this instance

exchange volumes of 10–20 ml/kg are generally used, with dialysate that can be either cooled or at room temperature

2. **Fill time, dwell time and drain time** Fluid removal rate is highest at the beginning of each exchange cycle, when the glucose concentration between the blood and the fresh dialysate solution is at its greatest. After a peak is reached, the removed volume falls as fluid is transported in the reverse direction, i.e. from the dialysis fluid back to the blood. If the dialysis solution is kept in the abdominal cavity long enough, the patient will gain rather than lose fluid

3. **Composition of the dialysate** Bicarbonate dialysate, or 1.36%, 2.27% or 3.86% glucose. The higher the concentration of glucose, the larger the osmotic pressure, resulting in a larger fluid removal. It is possible to use a combination of these different solutions, either by giving 50% of each for every cycle (use burette) or by alternating the different strengths so each is given only on alternate cycles.

4. **Heparin** (500 IU/l) is usually added to the dialysate to prevent fibrin formation and clotting in the catheter. Potassium may also be added, in order to maintain a normal serum potassium level.

Most PD performed in the paediatric intensive case unit (PICU) is continuous, and is maintained until the child is able to pass urine and the kidneys are functioning adequately.

 Aim to use the minimum concentration of glucose dialysate when possible – prolonged use of the 3.86% solution can result in sclerosis of the peritoneum, making further PD impossible.

Problems

Technical problems with PD are mostly related to catheter malfunction; the rigid Trocath catheter with a stylet has largely disappeared and surgically placed Tenckhoff catheters are reported to have fewer complications (Wong & Geary 1988, Huber et al 1994, Chadha et al 2000).

- If fill time takes longer than 10 min, it usually indicates catheter obstruction
- If less than 80% of the previous fill volume returns during the full drainage period, then drainage is inadequate.

Causes

- External kinks
- Fibrin or blood clot plugging
- Poor position or migration of catheter
- Obstruction by omentum
- Leaks around catheter site.

Action

- Reposition patient
- Alert medical colleagues, as catheter may benefit from careful flushing with sterile saline; abdominal X-ray will confirm position of catheter in abdomen
- Fibrin clotting may require urokinase infusion into catheter
- Leaks around catheter site will increase the risk of infection in addition to impairing the dialysis process; therefore medical staff may have to introduce new catheter.

Peritonitis remains a constant threat, especially if there has been a lot of manipulation of the catheter. The standard features of cloudy PD fluid require urgent attention (Warady 2000). Management may include antibiotics administered via the PD catheter. Removal of the catheter will necessitate sutures to close the skin and may need to be undertaken in theatre.

CONTINUOUS VENO-VENOUS HAEMOFILTRATION

Haemofiltration = ultrafiltration + convection + fluid replacement.
    Continuous veno–venous haemofiltration (CVVH) is the removal of fluid via a semipermeable membrane (haemofilter) using a circuit with a pump. The blood is obtained and returned to the venous circulation; this is an uninterrupted process.
    Indications for use of CVVH:

- When PD is contraindicated or has failed
- Hypervolaemia that does not require haemodialysis because of improving renal function (urea, creatinine and other electrolytes assessed)
- To ensure that adequate nutrition can be given in suitable volumes, to help decrease or prevent catabolism, and the equivalent volume can be removed.

CONTINUOUS VENO-VENOUS HAEMODIAFILTRATION (CVVHD)

Haemodiafiltration = ultrafiltration + convection + fluid replacement + diffusion.
    Continuous veno–venous haemodiafiltration (CVVHD) is the removal of excess fluid and biochemical waste products via a semipermeable membrane (haemofilter). Dialysis is performed by infusing dialysate fluid using a countercurrent flow through the haemofilter. The circuit has a pump. The blood is obtained and returned to the venous circulation; this is an uninterrupted process.
    Indications for the use of CVVHD:

- When PD is contraindicated or has failed
- To ensure that parenteral nutrition can be given in suitable volumes, to help decrease or prevent catabolism, ensuring that the equivalent volume can be removed

- When electrolytes are seriously deranged – particularly potassium
- In certain metabolic disorders, e.g. hyperammonaemia
- When child is not cardiovascularly stable enough to tolerate haemo-dialysis.

HAEMODIALYSIS

Haemodialysis = ultrafiltration + diffusion.

Haemodialysis is the removal of excess fluid and biochemical waste products via a semipermeable membrane (haemofilter). Dialysis is performed by infusing dialysate fluid using a countercurrent flow through the haemofilter. The circuit has a pump. The blood is obtained from and returned to the venous circulation.

Haemodialysis is an intermittent treatment; it can be used as a 'follow-on' treatment for children who, when critically ill, were receiving CVVHD, and whose condition is now stable enough to tolerate larger volumes of fluid and solute removal being undertaken on an intermittent, e.g. once daily, basis. In other cases its use, as opposed to CVVHD, is likely to depend on the haemodynamic stability of the PICU patient.

FLUIDS FOR CVVH/CVVHD

The purpose of predilution fluid is to achieve high ultrafiltration rates without additional risk of haemofilter thrombosis. There are a variety of types of replacement fluid manufactured for CVVH/D, which can be changed according to the patient's requirements and are categorised basically according to the inclusion/exclusion of potassium and buffer, which may be either bicarbonate or lactate. Other electrolytes may also need to be prescribed according to patient requirements.

The following are some examples:

- Potassium-free lactate-buffered fluid – Lactosol
- Potassium-free bicarbonate-buffered – Hemosol BO
- Potassium 4 mmol/l lactate-buffered – Hemolactol
- Potassium 4 mmol/l bicarbonate-buffered – Prismasol 4 (Gambro).

Hemosol BO is considered by some centres to be the fluid of choice for the majority of haemofiltered patients and the following points related to its use may be helpful:

- Buffered with bicarbonate (32 mmol/l) and does not require any additional bicarbonate infused into the patient
- Potassium free – add potassium according to guidelines. Never add more than 4 mmol/l of potassium
- The only relative contraindication to its use is metabolic alkalosis (pH > 7.5)
- This solution does not contain sufficient lactate to cause or mask hyperlactaemia and should still be used in these patients

To prepare Hemosol BO solution for use, the separate bicarbonate bag provided should be mixed in with the Hemosol BO as instructed by the manufacturer immediately before use (Evelina Children's Hospital PICU 2002).

 Do not add calcium or phosphate into this solution as it may precipitate. Always supplement Ca, Mg or phosphate directly to the patient (Evelina Children's Hospital PICU 2002).

 A predilution fluid should not contain more than 4 mmol/l of potassium regardless of how low the plasma potassium level may be. It is better to give IV potassium if hypokalaemia does not correct on haemofiltration (Evelina Children's Hospital PICU 2002).

PLASMA EXCHANGE

Plasma exchange is a treatment that is used to treat any disease that is plasma-mediated or plasma-borne, and any disease involving the immune system. The aim of the treatment is to remove autoantibodies, pathogenic immune complexes and inflammatory mediators. The treatment rapidly removes these substances, thereby reducing the effects of the disease processes.

Diseases that have been *treated* with plasma exchange include:

- Haemolytic uraemic syndrome (where there is neurological involvement)
- Guillain–Barré syndrome
- Systemic lupus erythematosus
- Renal transplant rejection
- Myasthenia gravis
- Henoch–Schönlein purpura.

A plasma filter is used for the procedure, and this removes the child's circulating plasma (albumin, antibodies and immune complexes, and clotting factors). During the procedure, the child is given albumin 4.5% to replace that removed. Fresh frozen plasma is also given to replace clotting factors lost. Therefore only the circulating antibodies and immune complexes are removed (Lowe 1997).

The PICU nurse's responsibilities include:

- Accurate measurement of fluid input and output
- Monitoring patient's haemodynamic status and altering fluid balance accordingly
- Prewarming replacement fluid and monitoring the patient's temperature
- Titration of heparin infusion to maintain optimal clotting times

- Regular assessment of blood gases and biochemistry
- Maintenance of asepsis with the catheter site and the blood circuit
- Maintenance of the blood circuit – acting as a 'troubleshooter'
- Source of information and reassurance to the patient and family.

Problems:

- Access difficulties
- Filter clotting
- Infections.

ANTICOAGULATION

The aim of anticoagulation is to prevent clotting of the extracorporeal circuit with minimal risk to the patient. Some authors believe that the filter should routinely be changed every 24 hours and that therefore the aim is to achieve its 24-hour lifespan (Ronco & Bellomo 2000).

Various methods of anticoagulation are used.

Heparin

Heparin acts by inhibiting the conversion of prothrombin to thrombin and neutralises the actions of thrombin. Some authors advise an initial bolus of heparin (maximum 50 IU/kg) at the time of connection to the extra-corporeal circuit followed by a continuous infusion of 0–30 IU/kg/h (Strazdins et al 2004); commonly the continuous infusion is administered at 5–10 IU/kg/h.

Record the amount of heparin infused hourly – this ensures that the heparin pump is infusing correctly and the correct dose is being given.

Some centres prefer to leave heparin infusing until treatment is discontinued – this ensures that patency of access is maintained after treatment is discontinued.

 You may need to give a bolus of heparin if blood products are administered, as the transfusion will increase the viscosity of the blood, which can lead to a decrease in the ultrafiltration, or solute removal and clotting problems may occur in the circuit.

Epoprostenol/prostacyclin

An infusion of prostacyclin may be used instead of heparin when the child has a low platelet count, to prevent or stop heparin-induced thrombocytopenia (Nevard & Rigden 1995).

Dose range: 1–2 ng/kg/min. In adults, dose ranges of 2–5 ng/kg/min have been widely used (Woodrow 1993, Kirby & Davenport 1996). Prosta-cyclin is a vasodilator and therefore may cause hypotension; however, doses of less than 5 ng/kg/min administered pre-filter are not usually associated with significant vasodilatation (Pearson 2002). Activated clotting time (ACT) monitoring is unhelpful because of prostacyclin's action in inhibiting platelet aggregation. Unlike heparin, boluses of prostacyclin should **not** be given when blood products are administered.

Citrate

Regional anticoagulation with citrate is favoured by some centres (Mehta et al 1991, Chadha et al 2002). Sodium citrate chelates ionised calcium necessary for the coagulation cascade and systemic anticoagulation is avoided by infusing calcium through a separate central line. The disadvantages include the possibility of various acid base and electrolyte disturbances including hypernatraemia, hypocalcaemia and metabolic alkalosis (Strazdins et al 2004).

Monitoring

Opinions vary as to the most effective way of monitoring anticoagulation; some centres believe that with patients with normal coagulation ACT should be used and aim for 120–180 s (Strazdins et al 2004). Others believe that ACT measurements are misleading and that partial thromboplastin time (PTT) should be used.

Although local guidelines must be adhered to, the following may be helpful:

- In patients with normal coagulation (international normalised ratio (INR) or PTT < 2.0 and platelets > 50):
  - Use a fixed rate of 10 IU/kg/h heparin
  - If PTT at 8 h > 2.0 reduce heparin dose to 5 IU/kg/h
  - If PTT persistently > 2.0 on 5 IU/kg/h **stop** anticoagulation
- In patients with coagulopathy (INR > 2.0, PTT > 2.0 or Plts < 50) or high risk of bleeding (defined as ongoing active bleeding/major bleed in last 48 h or surgery in last 24 h) **no anticoagulation**
- Do not use ACTs as a guide to degree of anticoagulation (inaccurate and misleading)
- If a filter clots in less than 24 h check that the Vas-Cath site is adequate (no kinking, etc.) (Evelina Children's Hospital PICU 2002).

The following should also be observed:

- Fibrin and clot deposition in venous bubble trap as clots build up in greater areas of stasis
- Rising venous pressure may indicate clot formation in the venous side of vascular access or venous bubble trap
- Rising transmembrane pressure (TMP) may indicate clot formation in the filter
- Darkening blood circuit may indicate clotting

- Continuous decrease in the rate of ultrafiltration
- Observe the haemofilter for clots, dark streaks or areas of gravity separation of the blood into plasma and cells.

Brief written observations on the condition of the circuit, recorded hourly on the appropriate chart, may be helpful.

 Patients may cool rapidly on CVVH as heat is lost across the haemofilter surface – monitor core temperature continuously and consider active warming measures. Some machines have the capacity to prewarm predilution fluid – use according to manufacturer's instructions and local policy.

Priming the circuit

When priming lines during setting up filter circuit, heparinised saline (5000 IU heparin to 1 litre 0.9% saline) is generally used. Where the circuit volume exceeds 10% of the child's extracorporeal blood volume and/or the child is anaemic, it is advisable to transfuse the volume of packed cells sufficient to correct the anaemia/provide the deficit in extracorporeal blood volume prior to starting haemofiltration. Some centres recommend priming the circuit with blood for neonates.

Checklist for CVVH/HD

1. Record patient weight
2. Place large bore Vas–Cath (preferably neck veins)
3. Confirm position of Vas–Cath prior to use
4. Select predilution fluid (add potassium according to guideline if potassium free fluid)
5. Blood prime if <10 kg
6. Select filter size according to weight
7. Choose optimal blood flow rate (BFR)
8. Set ultrafiltration rate (UFR)
9. Prescribe desired fluid balance (i.e. how much fluid to be removed per hour)
10. Anticoagulation as per regime
11. Monitor arterial/venous line pressure and TMP
12. Monitor patient temperature
13. Calculate filtration fraction, recirculation rates and sieving coefficient of urea
14. Change filter every 24 hours (adapted from Evelina Children's Hospital PICU 2002).

TROUBLESHOOTING CVVH/CVVHD: GENERAL REASONS FOR ALARMS

Alarm: Intermittent arterial pressure alarm.

Cause: Catheter intermittently sucking against vessel wall.

Action: Turn down pump speed, but not below three-quarters of the maximum rate; consider rotating the catheter 180°.
    Remember: the arterial sensor measures negative pressure. An increasingly negative arterial pressure reading indicates that it is becoming more difficult to pull blood out from the 'arterial' line. The catheter could be wedged against vessel/occluded/clotted.

Alarm: Arterial pressure alarm followed by venous pressure alarm.

Cause: Restriction of blood flow pre-pump causing arterial pressure alarm and stopping pump, causing venous pressure to drop and alarm.

Action: Correct, e.g. kinked line, poor position of catheter. Press venous pressure button to start blood pump and keep pressing until light goes out. If arterial pressure alarm comes on again, turn off blood pump and rotate catheter 180°. Restart pump.

Alarm: High venous pressure alarm.

Cause: Restriction of blood flow going back to the patient:
- Clotting in venous drip chamber
- Kinked line
- Poor catheter position.

Action: Check for kinks. Consider clots – try to wash back circuit, i.e. run saline through filter and venous bubble trap to aid visibility. Clots in venous line/filter? Need to change them.

Alarm: Air detector alarm and venous pressure alarm.

Cause: Level of blood in drip chamber fallen/frothing of blood in drip chamber.

Action: The pump will stop; raise the level in the drip chamber by removing air with a syringe. Restart pump.

The suggestions above are for general guidance only and are not intended to replace instructions in the operator's manual of individual machines.

RENAL DISEASE

Two renal diseases which may require the admission of a child to a PICU are nephrotic syndrome and haemolytic–uraemic syndrome.

Nephrotic syndrome

Nephrotic syndrome is a symptom complex characterised by oedema, marked proteinuria, hypercholesterolaemia and hypoalbuminaemia. Although there are many types of the disease, minimal change nephrotic syndrome is the most common in children.

The syndrome may be classified as primary (associated with a primary glomerular disease) or secondary (resulting from a wide variety of disease states or nephrotoxic agents).

- For unknown reasons the glomerular membrane, usually impermeable to large proteins, becomes permeable
- Protein, especially albumin, leaks through the membrane and is lost in the urine
- Plasma proteins decrease as proteinuria increases
- The colloidal osmotic pressure, which holds water in the vascular compartments, is reduced as a result of the decreased amount of serum albumin. This allows fluid to flow from the capillaries into the extracellular space, producing oedema. Accumulation of fluid in the interstitial spaces and peritoneal cavity is also increased by an overproduction of aldosterone, which causes retention of sodium. There is increased susceptibility to infection because of decreased gammaglobulin.

Management is aimed at:

- restoration or maintenance of adequate circulating blood volume and systemic perfusion
- maintenance of fluid and electrolyte balance
- minimising glomerular damage and maximising renal function
- ensuring patient comfort and preventing infection.

Most cases respond to steroid therapy, which appears to affect the basic disease process in addition to controlling the oedema. Those who are not steroid-responsive or who lose steroid responsiveness may respond to cytotic therapy (Pearson 2002).

 Urine specific gravity will be falsely elevated in the presence of proteinuria with the administration of osmotic diuretics. Urine osmolality is believed to be the best indicator of renal function because it reflects renal concentrating ability and is not affected by the presence of large molecules in the urine (Brunner & Suddarth 1991).

Haemolytic–uraemic syndrome

Haemolytic–uraemic syndrome (HUS) is the association of an acute haemolytic anaemia, thrombocytopenia and acute renal failure. This syndrome is one of the most common causes of acute renal failure in children. It often follows a gastrointestinal illness or, in older children, an upper respiratory illness.

Coxsackie viruses and, more commonly, *Escherichia coli* O157 have been isolated from HUS patients.

- The main site of injury is believed to be the endothelial lining of the small arteries and arterioles, particularly in the kidney
- The intravascular deposition of platelets and fibrin results in partial or complete occlusion of the small arterioles and capillaries in the kidney
- As a result of passing through these vessels, it is believed that erythrocytes are damaged, removed from the circulation by the spleen, and their life span reduced, resulting in a severe, progressive anaemia
- Thrombocytopenia may be present, possibly caused by the aggregation, consumption or destruction of platelets within the kidney
- HUS is associated with damage to the glomerular endothelial cells. As a result, renal blood flow and glomerular filtration rate can be reduced in a degree proportional to the glomerular injury
- Cortical necrosis may be produced by renal ischaemia, and renal tubular damage may be seen. While much of this damage is reversible, recurrences can occur or progressive renal failure may develop
- Central nervous system involvement may be evident. Irritability, seizures, abnormal posturing, hemiparesis or hypertensive encephalopathy may develop. It is believed that the development of neurological symptoms, particularly coma, is associated with a poor prognosis.

Management is aimed at:

- achieving and maintaining correct fluid and electrolyte balance
- blood transfusions as required
- treatment of anuria or oliguric renal failure may require peritoneal or haemodialysis
- management of hypertension – hypertension related to hypervolaemia can be managed with haemofiltration or dialysis
- if the child has bloody diarrhoea and/or abdominal distension with decreased gut motility, it may be necessary to be nil by mouth with the provision of parenteral nutrition
- recognition and treatment of any neurological complications
- informing and supporting the child and family (adapted from Hazinski 1992).

REFERENCES

Brunner L., Suddarth D.S. 1991 The Lippincott manual of pediatric nursing, 4th edn. Chapman & Hall, London

Chadha V, Warady B, Blowey D et al 2000 Tenckhoff catheters prove superior to Cook catheters in pediatric acute peritoneal dialysis. Am J Kidney Dis 35: 1111–1116

Chadha V, Garg U, Warady B, Alon U 2002 Citrate clearance in children receiving continuing venovenous renal replacement therapy. Pediatr Nephrol 17: 819–824

Evelina Children's Hospital PICU 2002 PICU haemofiltration manual. Unpublished. Guy's and St Thomas' NHS Foundation Trust, London

Hazinski M F (ed) 1992 Nursing care of the critically ill child, 2nd edn. C V Mosby, St Louis, MO

Huber R, Fuchshuber A, Huber P 1994 Acute peritoneal dialysis in preterm newborns and small infants: surgical management. J Pediatr Surg 29: 400–422

Kirby S, Davenport A 1996 Haemofiltration/dialysis treatment in patients with acute renal failure. Care Crit Ill 12(2): 54–58

Lowe R 1997 Introduction to Timbo Ward. Unpublished teaching package. Guy's and St Thomas' NHS Foundation Trust, London

Mehta R, McDonald B, Ward D 1991 Regional citrate anticoagulation for continuous arteriovenous hemodialysis: an update after 12 months. Contrib Nephrol 93: 210–214

Nevard CF, Rigden SP 1995 Haemofiltration in paediatric practice. Curr Paediatr 5: 14–16

Pearson G 2002 Handbook of paediatric intensive care. WB Saunders, Edinburgh

Ronco C, Bellomo R 2000 Continuous haemofiltration in acute renal failure. Lancet 356: 1442

Strazdins V, Watson A, Harvey B 2004 Renal replacement therapy for acute renal failure in children: European guidelines. Pediatr Nephrol 19: 199–207

Warady BA on behalf of the International Society of Peritoneal Dialysis Advisory Committee on Peritonitis Management in Pediatric Patients 2000 Consensus guidelines for the treatment of peritonitis in pediatric patients receiving peritoneal dialysis. Peritoneal Dialysis Int 20: 610–624

Woodrow P 1993 Resource package: Haemofiltration. Intens Crit Care Nurs 9: 95–107

Wong SN, Geary DF 1998 Comparison of temporary and permanent catheters for acute peritoneal dialysis. Arch Dis Childh 63: 827–831

LIVER DYSFUNCTION

5

The liver performs many functions, which can be divided into three general categories:

- **Metabolism** The liver metabolises carbohydrates, fats, proteins, drugs, hormones and bilirubin. It stores the end proteins, uses them to synthesise new proteins or releases them for excretion. The majority of plasma proteins (with the exception of gamma globulins) are formed by the hepatocytes, e.g. alpha and beta globulins, albumin, prothrombin and fibrinogen. Albumin is significant as it serves as a vehicle for substances such as drugs, bilirubin and hormones and plays a vital role in maintaining oncotic equilibrium. Clotting factors I, II, V, VII, IX and X are synthesised in the hepatocytes. Liver failure can be characterised by failure to synthesise these factors, resulting in coagulopathy. The liver also synthesises inhibitors of coagulation, further complicating the coagulopathy of liver disease as disseminated intravascular coagulation (DIC) may occur
- **Filtration** Kupffer cells make up approximately 10% of all cells in the liver. Their principal functions include phagocytes of particulate matter, detoxification of endotoxin, prolongation of the life of hepatocytes, secretion of mediators, regulation of hepatic microcirculation, processing of antigens, mediation of various immune responses and uptake, and catabolism of lipids and glycoproteins, including many enzymes
- **Storage** Although it usually holds about 600 ml of blood (in an adult), the liver can also contain large amounts during fluid shifts, vascular alterations or other conditions. It also stores vitamins and minerals. (Adapted from Siconolfi 1995)

The assessment of a paediatric liver disorder is based on the following:

- Clinical findings
- Biochemistry
- Imaging (Mowat 1994).

A variety of tests measure different aspects of liver failure (Table 5.1) – however, one enzyme, alanine transaminase (ALT), is a specific indicator of liver cell necrosis – most ALT elevations are caused by liver damage. In addition to this, INR is the best indicator of liver function.

Table 5.1 Liver function tests (adult American values have been replaced by commonly accepted British values)

Specific test	Normal range	Levels elevated because of:
Alanine transferase (ALT)	0–55 U/l	Hepatitis, hepatotoxic drugs, cholestasis
Alkaline phosphatase (ALP)	145–320 U/l	Biliary obstruction, primary liver tumour
Gamma glutamyl transferase (GGT)	8–78 U/l	Hepatitis, cirrhosis, cholestasis
Lactate dehydrogenase (LDH)	286–580 U/l	Myocardial infarction, haemolytic anaemia
Serum ammonia	< 40 µmol/l	Renal failure, hepatic encephalopathy, coma
Bilirubin – total	0–22 µmol/l	Hepatitis, jaundice, neonatal jaundice, obstruction of bile flow, infection
Prothrombin time (PT) or INR	0.8–1.1 s	Vitamin K deficiency, DIC, salicylate intoxication
Activated prothrombin time (APTT)	0.8–1.2 s	Clotting factor deficiencies, DIC
Fibrinogen	2.02–4.24 g/l	

Source: adapted and used with permission from *Nursing* 1995; 95(May): 41, © Springhouse Corporation/www.springnet.com.

ACUTE LIVER FAILURE

Aetiology in children is age-dependent. Most metabolic disorders and some specific infective agents cause liver failure in the neonatal period and infancy. In children older than 2, aetiologies are similar to adults; however, a large population are cryptogenic (Bhaduri & Vergani 1996).

Subgroups of hyperacute, acute and subacute liver failure reflect the different clinical patterns of the illness, aetiology and prognosis (Table 5.2). These universal classifications originate from O'Grady et al (1993) based on a retrospective analysis of 539 cases.

The above definitions can be applied in the paediatric population but do not necessarily encompass the complexity of the condition in the paediatric age group. In children, particularly during infancy, encephalopathy may appear late, if at all, and is an ominous sign. Mortality is high in paediatric patients with acute liver failure and neurological complications of encephalopathy and cerebral oedema are major contributors to mortality (Alper et al 1998). Acute liver failure may be the first presentation of an underlying metabolic disorder. A more appropriate definition for paediatrics is:

> a rare multisystem disorder in which severe impairment of liver
> function with or without encephalopathy occurs in association

Table 5.2 Classification of acute liver failure

	Interval of jaundice to encephalopathy	Cerebral oedema	Prognosis	Leading cause
Hyperacute	7 days	Common	Moderate	Virus A, B paracetamol
Acute	8–28 days	Common	Poor	Non A/B/C; drugs
Subacute	29 days–12 weeks	Poor	Poor	Non A/B/C; drugs

Source: adapted from O'Grady et al 1993.

with massive hepatic necrosis. In the absence of encephalopathy the severity of liver impairment is best assessed by the severity of coagulopathy (Bhaduri & Vergani 1996, p 349).

Encephalopathy

Encephalopathy and cerebral oedema is a frequent complication in adult patients and some paediatric patients. The cause of the encephalopathy is not clear; however, a wide range of neurotoxic properties accumulate in the circulation in liver failure. These substances can cross the blood–brain barrier and include ammonia, manganese, octanoate, aromatic amino acids and neuroactive medications, e.g. benzodiazepines. Ammonia accumulation in the brain causes adverse effects on excitatory and inhibitory neurotransmission, cerebral energy metabolism and expression of gene coding for key proteins in central nervous system function (Butterworth 2002).

In children, especially infants, encephalopathy is uncommon and an ominous sign. An incidence of a child with an international normalised ratio (INR) above 4 at any time is associated with a 92% mortality rate and is currently the criterion used for emergency listings, although each case is assessed individually. No specific diagnosis is possible before orthoptic liver transplantation (OLT) in 40–50% of cases, which should not delay the procedure. Neonates with a coagulopathy have a particularly bad prognosis (Lee 1993, Baker et al 1998, Riordan & Williams 1999).

CAUSES OF LIVER FAILURE

These include:

• Inherited/metabolic, e.g. Wilson's disease, galactosaemia
• Autoimmune diseases
• Infective, e.g. malaria, cytomegalovirus (CMV)
• Infiltrative, e.g. leukaemia
• Toxic or drug-related, e.g. paracetamol, cytotoxic drugs
• Ischaemic, e.g. due to sepsis/shock (Mowat 1994).

Table 5.3	Hepatic encephalopathy grading
Grade 0	Clinically normal mental status but minimal changes in memory, concentration, intellectual function and co-ordination
Grade 1	Mild confusion/anxiety, disturbed or reversal of sleep rhythm, shortened attention span, slowing of ability to perform mental tasks (simple addition or subtraction). In young children, irritability, altered sleep pattern, unexplained bursts of excessive crying.
Grade 2	Drowsiness, confusion, mood swings with personality changes, inappropriate behaviour, intermittent disorientation of time and place, gross deficit in ability to perform mental tasks. In young children, excessive sleepiness, inability to interact with or recognise parents, lack of interest in favourite toys and activities.
Grade 3	Pronounced confusion, delirious but arousable, persistent disorientation of time and place, hyperreflexia with a positive Babinski's sign.
Grade 4	Comatose with or without decerebrate or decorticate posturing, response to pain present (IVa) or no response to pain (IVb)

In the paediatric intensive care unit (PICU), liver failure may more commonly result as part of multiorgan failure in the critically ill child. In some diseases, however, the clinical presentation of liver failure can be unusual:

- Metabolic, e.g. Reye's syndrome
- Infections, e.g. hepatitis
- Toxic, e.g. phenytoin, aspirin
- Haemorrhagic.

Reye's syndrome is a multisystem disease characterised by a severe encephalopathy with a very high ammonia level, together with fatty degeneration and infiltration of the viscera (especially the liver) following recovery from a viral illness. Diagnosis is confirmed by liver biopsy.

THE JAUNDICED BABY

Unconjugated and conjugated hyperbilirubinaemia

Jaundice is caused by abnormally high levels of the pigment bilirubin in the blood (Fig. 5.1). There are two types of bilirubin – unconjugated and conjugated.

Most units have charts where the age/gestation of the infant is plotted, together with the weight and the unconjugated bilirubin level, in order to assess if phototherapy is indicated.

Kernicterus is yellow (bilirubin) staining of the basal ganglia in the brain of neonates with severe jaundice. Acidosis, neuronal dysfunction, alteration in the blood – brain barrier, hypercapnia and seizures are all thought to be contributing factors to the entry of bilirubin to the brain.

Fig. 5.1 The normal metabolism of bilirubin (with permission from McCance & Heuther 1992)

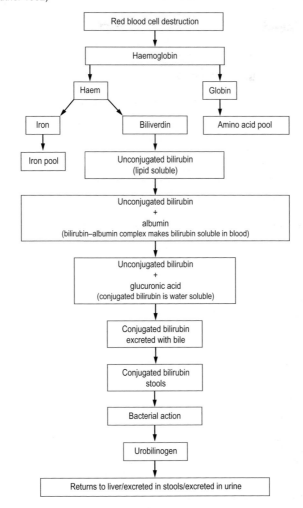

Phototherapy

Phototherapy is the use of blue/ultraviolet light on neonates, which causes bilirubin oxidation and destruction. The infant is kept unclothed to maximise the surface area exposed to the light, so appropriate measures are required to prevent heat loss (e.g. covered incubator). Protective patches are placed over the infant's eyes. Insensible water loss is increased during phototherapy and the fluid allowance will be increased accordingly, so accurate recording of fluid balance is important.

Unconjugated bilirubin

- Lipid-soluble
- High levels toxic to the brain – kernicterus
- Responds to phototherapy
- High levels can be caused by:
  - Excessive production of blood cells, i.e. red blood cells breaking up too quickly
  - Immature liver, which cannot conjugate bilirubin quickly enough – cause of jaundice frequently seen in infants
  - Abnormality in the liver preventing the conjugation of bilirubin – rare.

Conjugated bilirubin

- Water-soluble
- Excreted in stool/urine/bile
- High levels can be caused by:
  - Obstruction to flow of bile from liver, e.g. biliary atresia
  - Abnormally small and/or reduced number of bile ducts inside the liver
  - Liver disease causing damage to liver cells, e.g. infection, genetic disease.

A 'split' bilirubin level test measures serum levels of unconjugated and conjugated bilirubin. Jaundice in any baby aged 14 days or over must always be investigated.

Sengstaken tube

A Sengstaken tube may be used in a child with chronic liver failure who has oesophageal varices. It is a rubber tube that has two inflatable balloons at the lower end, one of which when inflated exerts direct pressure on the oesophagus while the other maintains the position of the tube. Correctly positioned in the oesophagus, this tube can stop the bleeding of varices by applying direct pressure of the inflated balloon on the submucosa. This technique is only usually undertaken by a senior member of the surgical/intensivist medical team under intravenous (IV) sedation.

Goals of management

The goals of management of liver failure are as follows:

- Treat primary hepatic injury, e.g. coma, hypoglycaemia and coagulopathy. Hypoglycaemia may be profound, requiring 25–50% IV dextrose solutions to maintain a blood sugar of 4 mmol/l. Maintenance fluid should not be stopped, even for a short period of time
- Prevent secondary injury e.g. pulmonary oedema, cerebral oedema, shock, renal dysfunction, infection, pancreatitis and death.

Management may therefore include multisystem support, including the following:

- Ventilation
- Fluid, electrolyte and coagulation correction and monitoring
- Management of cerebral oedema
- Pharmacological implications – compromised metabolic and excretory functions result in extended half-lives of many drugs
- Haemodialysis or haemodiafiltration to support renal failure or to reduce ammonia levels in hyperammonaemia (Reye's syndrome/inborn errors of metabolism).

HEPATORENAL SYNDROME

This refers to unexplained renal failure in patients with liver disease or those undergoing surgery for biliary tract obstruction. The kidneys are normal. Although frequently overloaded, there is often intravascular depletion. This leads to a reduced renal output, an elevated urea and creatinine and a low serum sodium. Management includes a fluid bolus, use of diuretics and measurement of CVP (Stack & Dobbs 2004).

In the event that liver failure is not part of overall multiorgan failure, extensive laboratory investigations may be necessary to find the cause and to determine whether any specific treatment is indicated. There is currently no rescue therapy in the event of severe liver failure. Transplantation is the only life-saving procedure and centres that perform this surgery have certain criteria for assessing whether or not it is indicated. Transfer to specialist centres should therefore be arranged in this instance, together with the incorporation of their recommendations for the management of the child prior to and during transfer (De Jaeger & Lacroix 1997).

REFERENCES

Alper G, Jarjour IT, Reyes JD et al 1998 Outcome of children with cerebral oedema caused by fulminant hepatic failure. Pediatr Neurol 18: 299–304

Baker A, Dhawan A, Heaton N 1998 Who needs a liver transplant? (New disease specifications.) Arch Dis Childh 79:460–464

Bhaduri B, Vergani GM 1996 Fulminant liver hepatic failure: paediatric aspects. Semin Liver Dis 16: 349–354

Butterworth R 2002 Prevention and management of hepatic encephalopathy. Improved outcome with extracorporeal support. Insert for intensive care physicians. Intens Care Med 28: 11

De Jaeger A, Lacroix J 1997 Hepatic failure. In: Singh NC (ed) Manual of pediatric critical care. WB Saunders, Philadelphia, PA

Lee W 1993 Acute liver failure. N Engl J Med 329: 1862–1870

McCance KL, Heuther S 1992 Pediatric gastrointestinal disorders. In: Hazinski MF Nursing care of the critically ill child, 2nd edn. CV Mosby, St Louis, MO

Mowat AP 1994 Liver disorders in childhood, 3rd edn. Butterworth Heinemann, Oxford

O'Grady J, Schalm S, Williams R 1996 Acute liver failure: redefining the syndromes. Lancet 342: 275

Riordan SM, Williams R 1999 Cause and prognosis in acute liver failure Liver Transpl Surg 5: 86–89

Siconolfi LA 1995 Clarifying the complexity of liver function tests. Nursing May: 39–44

Stack C, Dobbs P 2004 Essentials of paediatric intensive care. Greenwich Medical, London

Useful websites

www.bspghan.org.uk
www.aasld.org

NEUROLOGY ASSESSMENT AND MANAGEMENT

6

In the paediatric intensive care unit (PICU) environment, the nurse is likely to encounter a variety of causes of neurological deficit, requiring careful assessment and management.

DISORDERS CAUSING COMA IN CHILDREN

These include:

- Hypoxic–ischaemic brain injury following respiratory or circulatory failure
- Epileptic seizures
- Trauma
  - Intracranial haemorrhage, cerebral oedema
- Infections
  - Meningitis, encephalitis
- Poisoning
- Metabolic
  - Renal/hepatic failure, Reye's syndrome, hypoglycaemia, ketoacidosis, hypothermia, hypercapnia
- Vascular lesions
  - Bleeding, arteriovenous malformations, arterial or venous thrombosis

(adapted from Advanced Life Support Group 2005).

ASSESSMENT

A rapid measure of the level of consciousness can be recorded using the AVPU scale:

A   Alert
V   responds to Voice
P   responds to Pain (= GCS ≤ 8)
U   Unresponsive

(Advanced Life Support Group 2005).

A variety of neurological assessment tools are in use – many are derivatives of the Glasgow Coma Scale (Teasdale & Jennett 1974) or the

Fig 6.1   Example of neurological assessment charts: Glasgow Coma Scale and Children's Glasgow Coma Scale (under 5 years).

Glasgow Coma Scale (4–15 years)		Child's Glasgow Coma Scale (<4 years)	
Response	Score	Response	Score
Eye opening		**Eye opening**	
Spontaneously	4	Spontaneously	4
To verbal stimuli	3	To verbal stimuli	3
To pain	2	To pain	2
No resoponse to pain	1	No response to pain	1
Best motor response		**Best motor response**	
Obeys verbal command	6	Spontaneous or obeys verbal command	6
Localises to pain	5	Localises to pain or withdraws to touch	5
Withdraws from pain	4	Withdraws from pain	4
Abnormal flexion to pain (decorticate)	3	Abnormal flexion to pain (decorticate)	3
Abnormal extension to pain (decerebrate)	2	Abnormal extension to pain (decerebrate)	2
No response to pain	1	No response to pain	1
Best verbal response		**Best verbal response**	
Orientated and converses	5	Alert, babbbles, coos, words to usual ability	5
Disorientated and converses	4	Less than usual words spontaneous irritable cry	4
Inappropriate words	3	Cries only to pain	3
Incomprehensible sounds	2	Moans to pain	2
No response to pain	1	No response to pain	1

Adelaide Scale (Simpson & Reilly 1982). The need for the tool to be age-appropriate, i.e. for the neurological immaturity of the child to be taken into consideration, has been recognised, in order to improve the accuracy and validity of the assessment.

An example of an age-appropriate chart is illustrated in Figure 6.1.

GUIDELINES FOR NEUROLOGICAL ASSESSMENT

- The chart should be used as part of an overall assessment, including vital signs, assessment of fontanelle, if appropriate, and the child's reaction to his/her surroundings and, in particular, to family/caregivers
- Care must be taken to ensure that the pain application, where required, is appropriate and applied for a sufficient length of time to allow the

best response to be elicited – until the patient responds, or a minimum of 15 and maximum of 30 seconds is recommended (Lower 2002).

- The effects of drugs that are being administered or have been administered must be acknowledged
- Continuity of interpretation of neurological observations is improved if, during handover between shifts, a joint neurological assessment is executed, e.g. agreement on pupil size
- A careful explanation of all procedures to be used during a neurological assessment must be given to relatives/visitors in order to minimise distress.

Eye opening

The ability to obey commands is dependent upon the age and compliance of the child.

If the child does not open her eyes spontaneously, assess her response to speech by calling her name, first quietly and then loudly should there be no initial response. If the child is of preschool age and above, ask her to open her eyes. In order to elicit the best response, ask the child's parents, if present, to call her name. If there is no response use a graded sequence of stimulation as recommended by Lower (2002) – shout, shake, pain. The interpretation of 'shake' is intended as a rousing stimulus rather than an actual physical shaking action, prior to the application of a pain stimulus (details below under motor response) to a child who may simply be drowsy.

In order to assess pupils, unless eyes are open, open both carefully and assess size of pupils together – it is easier to see differences when both are viewed simultaneously. The use of a pupil size chart beside the child's face can promote accurate measurement of pupil size. Consider also the lighting in the child's bed space; if it is either very bright or dimmed, this could affect the pupil size when assessed. Interpretation can also differ between assessing individuals.

Each pupil's response to light is recorded appropriately with a + or − sign, and an H for hippus response, which occurs when the pupil constricts then dilates to light. Note whether the pupils respond briskly or sluggishly. If in doubt, get a colleague to check.

Eyes that are closed by swelling can be indicated by C − if the chart you are using does not specify the above, you could formulate a 'key' for clarification. Note also the position of the pupils, e.g. they may be divergent, or 'sunsetting' in appearance – pupils resemble a setting sun because of downward deviation caused by pressure on cranial nerve III, the oculomotor nerve.

Verbal response

Charts will vary in the age-appropriateness of this category. In the charts shown, while 'orientated and converses' indicates the best response from the 5-year-old, 'babbles, coos, words to usual ability' is the best response from babies and children under this age. 'Cries to pain' is an appropriate response in the youngest infants – 0–6 months. Again, involve the parents where possible and take into consideration the child's own stage of development. Has the child reached developmental milestones or are there known delays/deficits? The inability to produce a verbal response because of an endotracheal or tracheostomy tube is documented as T.

Motor response

If the child obeys commands, e.g. by squeezing your fingers or wriggling his toes when asked, he may also be able to lift his hands and feet off the bed, or push against you with them. This enables you to assess any differences in strength/weakness between the child's left and right sides. Ensure that the *best* motor response is charted, as well as differences; involve parents where possible.

Painful stimuli should be central to avoid eliciting a spinal or reflex response. This approach may include:

- Pressing the superior orbital ridge
- Sternal rub
- Trapezius squeeze (children aged 5 years and above only, because there is insufficient development of muscle before this age).

Consider other injuries/surgical procedures, e.g.

- Avoid orbital ridge if facial injuries present
- Avoid sternal rub if chest injuries/surgery.

As stated above, administer for a sufficient time to allow the best response to be elicited – until the patient responds, or a minimum of 15 and maximum of 30 seconds (Lower 2002).

The application of a peripheral pain stimulus is appropriate on certain occasions, e.g. when all limbs except one respond to central pain stimulus and it is necessary to test whether that limb is capable of moving. Press a pencil against a nail bed for the time as stated previously and monitor the reaction (Lower 2002).

A child aged 6–24 months is deemed capable of localising pain but from 0–6 months the maximum response is flexion to pain. In contrast to appropriate flexion there is also abnormal posturing:

- Decorticate posturing: abnormal flexion of limbs to centre of body and rigid extension of legs
- Decerebrate posturing: rigid extension of all four limbs.

Consider also cough and gag reflexes (endotracheal tube/tracheostomy suctioning and using Yankauer at back of throat, respectively, could be used to test these).

- Posturing: Does the child appear to move normally or abnormally?
- Motor responses: Any change is likely to be on the opposite side of the problem

Table 6.1 Summary of pupil changes

Pupil size and reactivity	Cause
Small reactive pupils	Metabolic disorders
	Medullary lesion
Pin-point pupils	Metabolic disorders
	Narcotic/organophosphate ingestion*
Fixed midsized pupils	Midbrain lesion
Fixed dilated pupils	Hypothermia
	Severe hypoxia
	Barbiturates (late sign)
	During and post seizure
	Anticholinergic drugs
Unilateral dilated pupil	Rapidly expanding ipsilateral lesion
	Tentorial herniation
	Third nerve lesion
	Epileptic seizures

* Pupil constriction can also be caused by prescribed drugs, e.g. morphine/fentanyl, in addition to ingestion.
Source: with permission from Advanced Life Support Group 2005.

- Pupillary responses: Changes usually occur on the same side as the lesion; for example, if a brain tumour is on the left side, the pupil changes will be on the left and the motor changes will be on the right.

Pupil constriction can be caused by drugs, e.g. fentanyl or morphine. Bilaterally dilated pupils may indicate hypoxia or be due to drugs, e.g. atropine.

A suddenly dilated pupil, or unequal pupils, is a warning sign of serious problems.

The hippus response is where the pupils can not sustain the constriction to light and redilate. Hippus response may be normal if pupils are observed under high magnification but it is also observed at the beginning of pressure on cranial nerve III and can be associated with early transtentorial herniation.

A suddenly dilated pupil (which if fixed can be referred to as a child 'blowing' a pupil), or unequal pupils should serve as a serious warning sign, requiring immediate medical assessment and probably a computed tomography (CT) scan.

IDENTIFICATION AND MANAGEMENT OF RAISED INTRACRANIAL PRESSURE

The Monro–Kellie doctrine observes that the total intracranial volume cannot expand as the skull is a rigid structure that contains a finite intracranial volume. The intracranial pressure is determined by the total intracranial volume and intracranial compliance (the change in pressure resulting from a change in volume). Skull sutures are not fixed in infancy and can expand to accommodate *gradual* increases in intracranial volume but not *acute* increases – therefore even in infancy intracranial volume is relatively constant.

Intracranial contents include:

- Brain: occupies approximately 80% of intracranial space
- Blood – cerebral blood volume (CBV): occupies 7–10% of the total intracranial volume
- Cerebrospinal fluid (CSF): occupies 7–10% of the total intracranial volume.

Intracranial volume = Brain volume + Blood volume + CSF volume.

If the volume of any of the intracranial contents increases without a commensurate and compensatory decrease in the volume of other substances in the intracranial vault, intracranial pressure will rise.

The relationship between intracranial pressure and cerebral perfusion pressure

The normal range of intracranial pressure (ICP) is:

- Infants: 1.6–6 mmHg
- Young children: 3–7 mmHg
- Older children/adults: 10–15 mmHg (Chitnavis & Polkey 1998).

Transient increases can be caused by coughing or by moving from a standing to a reclining position, which causes an increase in venous pressure as a result of compensation mechanisms (below). Once the limits of these mechanisms have been reached, significant increases in ICP are seen. The optimum range of ICP for children with severe head injury is not clear; however, it is suggested that ICP should be kept below 20 mmHg (Hazinski 1992; Shann & Henning 2003).

Cerebral perfusion pressure (CPP) is the difference between the mean systemic blood pressure and the intracranial pressure:

CPP = Mean systemic arterial pressure (MAP) − Intracranial pressure (ICP).

An adequate CPP is:

- Neonate >30 mmHg
- 1 month–1 year >50 mmHg
- 1 year–10 years >60 mmHg
- More than 15 years >70 mmHg (Shann & Henning 2003).

CPP will fall if the MAP falls, if the mean ICP rises or if both occur simultaneously. The CPP can be maintained despite a rise in ICP if the MAP rises with it. This may or may not be associated with effective cerebral perfusion.

If there is high ICP and high CPP there must be high blood pressure.
Look for the cause of the high blood pressure, e.g. pain, and treat it.
Do not give antihypertensive drugs (Shann & Henning 2003).

Causes of raised ICP

- Trauma, e.g. road traffic accident/blow to head
- Encephalitis
- Cerebral oedema, e.g. infection/trauma/renal problems/sodium imbalance/hypoxia
- Tumours
- CSF alteration
  - Increased production
  - Decreased absorption
  - Pathway obstruction
- Cerebrovascular alterations
  - Increased blood pressure
  - Vein of Galen (congenital abnormality where artery joins veins in skull)
  - Sodium imbalances.

Compensatory mechanisms

When CPP is altered, cerebral blood flow (CBF) is maintained by a compensation mechanism called cerebral autoregulation. When MAP decreases, cerebral vasodilatation occurs, with a large increase in CBV and ICP; when MAP increases, cerebral vasoconstriction occurs with a reduction in CBV and ICP.

- **Respiratory**
  - **High $P\text{CO}_2$** → vasodilation → *Raised* ICP
  - **Low $P\text{CO}_2$** → vasoconstriction → *Drop* in ICP
  - **Low $P\text{O}_2$** → vasodilation → *Raised* ICP
  - **Low pH** → vasodilation → *Raised* ICP
- **CSF** Can be displaced into spinal canal if temperature is high
- **Temperature** For every 1°C rise in body temperature, cerebral metabolism may rise by up to 19%, leading to a rise in ICP (Fisher 1997)
- **Stimulation** Stress → systemic vasoconstriction → blood pressure (BP) + CBF increased → Raised ICP.

Once the limits of compensation have been reached, a further increase in intracranial volume will result in a rise in ICP. Progressive small rises in intracranial volume will produce progressively greater rises in ICP.

Clinical signs and symptoms

A child with raised ICP may demonstrate an alteration in the following:

- Level of consciousness: likely to deteriorate
- Pupil reaction: unequal/unreactive/dilated
- Heart rate: decreasing
- Blood pressure: increasing
- Respiratory rate/pattern: slower and irregular
- Motor activity/reflexes/development of abnormal posturing: decorticate (flexion) or decerebrate (extension)
- Response to pain (demonstrating flaccidity).

The child may complain of a headache, or develop nausea and vomiting.

In some instances, Cushing's triad – hypertension/bradycardia/apnoea – may occur. (This is a late sign.)

X-rays, a CT scan or a magnetic resonance imaging (MRI) scan may be taken in order to assist with the assessment of the child's condition.

Management

The goals of managing raised ICP are as follows:

1. Ensure effective cerebral perfusion through the maintenance of good systemic perfusion and control of intracranial pressure
2. Preserve cerebral function
3. Prevent secondary insults to the brain.

Intubation and mechanical ventilation should be undertaken for the following:

- Coma – GCS $\leq$ 8 (= AVPU scale at P)
- Loss of protective laryngeal reflexes
- Ventilatory insufficiency – hypoxaemia, hypercapnia
- Spontaneous hyperventilation causing $P\text{CO}_2$ less than 3.5 kPa
- Respiratory arrhythmia

Hyperventilation and $P\text{CO}_2$: General evidence suggests that the $P\text{CO}_2$ should be kept within the lower end of the normal range (4.5–5.5 kPa). While hypocapnia produces a reduction in ICP and an increase in CPP, it also reduces CBF, to the extent of causing ischaemia (Stringer et al 1993, Skippen et al 1997). While prophylactic hyperventilation should be avoided, some suggest that mild hypercapnia – $P\text{CO}_2$ of 4–4.5 kPa – may be beneficial where raised ICP is refractory to sedation, analgesia, paralysis and hyperosmolar therapy. Aggressive hyperventilation may be useful for brief periods where there is an acute neurological deterioration or impending coning – usually while another management option is being organised.

Blood pressure: Monitor closely; maintain within normal range for the child or slightly hypertensive to maintain adequate CPP and counteract raised ICP (White et al 2001). In recent studies comparing it with dopamine, noradrenaline (norepinephrine) has been shown to augment cerebral perfusion and increase flow velocity in a predicable manner (Johnston et al 2004) and it is considered by some to be the vasoactive drug of choice.

Fluids and electrolytes: The importance of maintaining a good BP, CVP and CPP is balanced by the need to fluid-restrict (50–60% of full maintenance – opinions vary) and keep the child slightly dehydrated, causing high normal ranges in serum osmolality and serum sodium – alleviates cerebral oedema and reduces ICP. 0.9% saline is generally the fluid of choice. Ensure blood glucose is kept within normal range – insulin infusion may be necessary in some cases. Check and correct calcium, magnesium, potassium and PO_4.

Hyperosmolar therapy: Mannitol is an osmotic diuretic, i.e. it produces an acute and transient rise in intravascular osmolality, resulting in a shift of free water from the interstitial and cellular spaces to the intravascular space. This free water is then eliminated by the kidneys; observe urine output to monitor effect. *Dose*: 0.25–0.5 g/kg IV, providing serum osmolality is no greater than 320 mosmol to prevent risk of renal failure (Shann & Henning 2003). May be repeated 6-hourly if needed. There is a risk of reverse osmotic shift in damaged brain tissue.

Hypertonic (3%) saline has an osmotic effect in addition to anti-inflammatory properties and regulates neutrophil–endothelial cell interactions (Khanna et al 2000, Kamat et al 2003). *Dose*: 3 ml/kg is given in some centres.

Position: General evidence recommends:

- Midline – nose – sternum – umbilicus (Singh 1997)
- 30° head up-tilt (Feldman et al 1992)
- Support neck laterally – if spinal collar in situ ensure it is not too tight and thus impeding venous drainage
- Placing central venous lines in either the subclavian or internal jugular veins should be undertaken with caution as this may obstruct venous drainage and thus increase ICP
- Avoid extreme hip flexion – increases intrathoracic pressure and thus ICP

Noise reduction: Sudden loud noises can cause a startle reflex – associated rise in ICP.

- Monitors, alarms, telephones – try to silence promptly
- Prevent people talking negatively/airing their concerns about child's condition/accident/prognosis near the bedspace – may cause anxiety and subsequent rise in ICP (Schinner et al 1995).

Drugs: Analgesia and sedation are used to manage noxious and painful stimuli and to facilitate effective ventilatory support:

- Morphine/fentanyl
- Consider giving lidocaine via ETT; 2% at 1 mg/kg not more than 6-hourly before endotracheal tube (ET) suction has been shown be effective in reducing ICP spikes during ET suction (Dee & Park 2003)
- Paralysis, e.g. vecuronium infusion. It is suggested that neuromuscular blocking (paralysing) agents reduce ICP by a variety of mechanisms including a reduction in airway and intrathoracic pressure with facilitation of cerebral venous outflow and by the prevention of shivering, posturing or breathing against the ventilator (Hsiang et al 1994). Risks include the masking of seizures, which can be addressed by continuous EEG monitoring
- Antacids until enterally fed
- Barbiturates, e.g. thiopental, reduce ICP via a reduction in cerebral metabolic rate (by about 50% – Piatt & Schiff 1984) and resultant decrease in CBF and blood volume (Singh 1997). Hypotension is a common side effect and inotropic support may be required. EEG monitoring may be useful as near-maximum reduction in cerebral metabolism and CBF occurs at burst suppression.

 Although propofol is still used in some centres in the UK, continuous infusion of propofol for either sedation or the management of refractory intracranial hypertension in infants and children with severe traumatic brain injury is not recommended (Center for Drug Administration and Research 2001).

Temperature: Hyperthermia is associated with an increase in damage following brain injury by various mechanisms, including increasing cerebral metabolism, inflammation, lipid peroxidation, cell death and acute seizures. The ideal temperature is the subject of much debate but is generally 34–35°C.

- The prevention and aggressive treatment of fever and iatrogenic hyperthermia after head injury is emphasised (Singh 1997)
- Cooling to 35° to reduce metabolic demands and provide a degree of neuroprotection in patients with persistently raised ICP is advocated by some authors (Shiozaki et al 1998).

Care

- Staggering versus clustering – assess child and plan care accordingly
- Minimal handling
- Minimal physio/suctioning

- Avoid constipation/full bladder
- Avoid rapid changes in position
- Use log rolling to maintain alignment and prevent exacerbation of neck or spinal injury
- Consider bolus of sedation and informing child of all activities prior to carrying them out.

Monitoring

- Heart rate and rhythm
- BP and CVP
- ICP and CPP
- S_aO_2 and continuous $ETCO_2$
- Temperature
- Fluid balance
- Neuro assessment.

INTRACRANIAL PRESSURE MONITORING

ICP monitoring is a valuable addition to the clinical assessment of the patient. It is extremely helpful in the evaluation of trends in the patient's condition, particularly in response to therapy. ICP measurements should always be interpreted in conjunction with the patient's clinical appearance.

Two methods of monitoring ICP are:

- **Ventricular pressure monitoring** A catheter is inserted through a burr hole in the skull into the lateral ventricle and is attached to a fluid-filled (or fibreoptic) monitoring system
- **Subarachnoid screw pressure monitoring** The subarachnoid screw is inserted through a burr hole in the skull and attached to a fluid-filled (or fibreoptic) monitoring system, e.g. Camino bolt.

NB. Fibreoptic catheters are zeroed before they are placed, but fluid systems require zeroing on a daily or shift basis, with the transducer being levelled at the outer aspect of the eye.

Hourly charting of intracranial pressure on an appropriate chart should record the following:

1. The average number ICP that hour (the number used to calculate the CPP)
2. The highest peak ICP observed that hour.

This method makes it possible to accurately record trends in the ICP.

Once ICP is stable, there should be a gradual return to normal care, i.e.:

- Increase fluids
- Decrease ventilation

- Stop paralysis
- Decrease sedation
- Continue neurological assessment
- Continue to normalise care until extubation is possible.

Cerebrospinal fluid

CSF is mainly produced by the choroid plexuses in the lateral, third and fourth ventricles. From these production sites, the CSF fills the ventricular system and follows a pathway incorporating the subarachnoid space.

CSF flows over and around the brain and spinal cord, providing buoyancy and support and maintaining the constant chemical composition of the extracellular fluid in which the central nervous system metabolic activity occurs. Absorption of CSF into the venous circulation is via the arachnoid villi, which act as one-way valves and are located in the superior sagittal sinus.

CSF is produced at an approximate rate of:

- 20 ml/h in adults
- 5–10 ml/h in toddlers
- 3–5 ml/h in infants (Evans 1987).

CSF is made up of:

- White cells
- Water
- Oxygen
- Carbon dioxide
- Protein
- Glucose
- Sodium
- Potassium
- Chloride.

Indications for cerebrospinal fluid drainage

Extraventricular drainage diverts CSF from the ventricles in the brain when the normal physiological mechanisms are unable to do so. It can be used:

- to monitor intraventricular pressure and output of CSF
- to divert CSF that contains bacteria or blood
- in the emergency treatment of a malfunctioning internal shunt and hydrocephalus
- to control ventricular pressure.

Hydrocephalus

This is the result of an increase of CSF within the cranial vault, which causes ventricular dilatation. Types:

- Communicating hydrocephalus: occurs when the arachnoid villi are obstructed and unable to reabsorb the CSF, e.g. in subarachnoid haemorrhage
- Non-communicating hydrocephalus: caused by an obstruction in the flow of CSF within the ventricular system; causes include congenital malformation/tumour (Allen 1993).

Treatment

To treat hydrocephalus, a temporary or permanent ventricular shunt is surgically inserted to divert CSF.

A temporary shunt is a straight, silastic ventricular catheter, usually placed in the right lateral ventricle through a burr hole made in the parasagittal region of the skull, just anterior to the right coronal suture. The catheter is then attached directly to drainage tubing by an inter-locking connector that has an access port. This type of set up is called a simple extraventricular drain.

A permanent shunt is usually in the form of an internal ventriculo-peritoneal shunt, where the CSF is drained from the ventricles as above but is then tunnelled under the scalp, neck and chest wall to the abdomen, ending in the peritoneal cavity, where the draining CSF is absorbed (Birdsall & Grief 1990).

Extraventricular drains

Several systems are available; generally a measuring chamber is posi-tioned to drain CSF at a set pressure through the attached drainage system. Refer to local policies for specific management.

COMMON DIAGNOSTIC TESTS

Electroencephalography

The electroencephalograph (EEG) is a recording of the electrical activity arising from different areas of the brain.

These areas of activity can be quantified, localised and compared with normal EEGs for the patient's age to assist in the diagnosis of seizure activity or central nervous system injury or dysfunction. An isoelectric (flat) EEG in a non-sedated, non-hypothermic patient is one of the criteria used to confirm brain death.

An EEG is performed using electrodes placed on specific areas of the scalp – the number of these and their positioning depends on the specific machine used.

Computed tomography scan

Computed axial tomography consists of a series of X-rays that are analysed and reconstructed by a computer to produce cross-sectional images. In these circumstances, the X-ray pictures of the skull will produce cross-sectional images of the intracranial contents. The images produced by the scan allow differentiation of intracranial spaces and normal grey/white matter.

The CT scan is a reliable, painless and non-invasive method of visualising a variety of neurological disorders, including space-occupying lesions, haematomas, haemorrhages, hydrocephalus and brain abscesses.

> A higher radiation dose is used for CT than for conventional X-rays, but the value of this test is believed to outweigh this risk.

> If an intracranial lesion is identified, e.g. an extradural haematoma, the child will need urgent transfer to a neurosurgical centre. The referring centre should transport the child to avoid delay.

Magnetic resonance imaging scan

Magnetic resonance imaging (MRI) is the application of a strong external magnetic field around the patient, which causes rotation of the cell nuclei in a predictable direction at a predictable speed. The result of the rotation of the nuclei is a resonant image that is extremely well defined and enables the visualisation of soft tissues better than any other non-invasive device (Hazinski 1992). It is particularly valuable for visualisation of tumours, shunts and tissue or organ thicknesses. The scan also enables detailed visualisation of areas of spinal cord compression following trauma.

Both CT and MRI scans can take up to 30 min to complete, depending on the area that is scanned. As the patient needs to be completely still, it is important that the child is adequately sedated, paralysed if appropriate and monitored throughout the procedure.

A contrast medium may be administered intravenously, to assist in clarifying areas being examined.

The cerebral function analysing monitor (CFAM)

The electroencephalogram, or EEG, is a recording of the electrical activity within the brain. By recording this activity and then analysing it, valuable information can be obtained to assist diagnosis of seizure activity or central nervous system injury/dysfunction.

Different institutions have their own methods of obtaining continuous EEG recordings of the critically ill child.

FITTING

Fits (seizures) are sudden, abnormal discharges of cerebral neurons (BMJ 1997). They may be generalised (activity spread through the subcortical area, bilateral tonic–clonic activity possibly associated with loss of consciousness) or focal (activity localised in a small area of the cerebral cortex, unilateral tonic–clonic activity).

- **Tonic phase** Rigidity of muscles due to spasm
- **Clonic phase** Convulsive jerking movements, commonly of limbs and trunk.

Clinical signs of fitting may include the following:

- Changes in:
  - Blood pressure
  - Heart rate
  - Respiratory pattern
- Convulsions
- Cyanosis.

Commonly, specific charts are used to document episodes of fitting, where the following details are recorded:

- Description of the abnormal movements, e.g. smacking lips followed by repeated jerking of right arm
- Duration
- Whether self-resolving or, if medication was required, which drugs were administered and their effect.

It would also be beneficial to record whether the fits were spontaneous or triggered by an intervention, e.g. someone touching or moving the child.

 As abnormal movements do not necessarily constitute fits, **write what you see** to prevent inaccurate interpretation.

When an intubated child has been paralysed and sedated, clinical signs of fitting can be masked; the use of EEG monitoring in these circumstances can be valuable.

Causes of fitting

- Structural lesions, e.g.
  - Cerebral infarction
  - Tumour
  - Haematoma
  - Abscess
- Infection
  - Systemic
  - CNS
  - Encephalitis/meningitis
  - High-grade pyrexia
- Toxic ingestion
- Metabolic disorders
- Head trauma
- Seizure disorders, e.g. epilepsy
- Hypoxic–ischaemic encephalopathy.

Status epilepticus

This occurs either when a fit lasts for longer than 30 minutes or when successive seizures occur so frequently that the patient does not recover fully between them.

Status epilepticus can be fatal – death may be due to:

- Complications of the convulsion, such as obstruction of the airway or aspiration of vomit
- Overmedication
- Underlying disease process.

Injury to the brain during status epilepticus occurs as a result of one or more of the following:

- Direct injury from repetitive neuronal discharge
- Systemic complications of the convulsions, especially hypoxia from airway obstruction and later acidosis when systemic hypotension occurs
- The underlying disease process.

The most common causes of status epilepticus in children are:

- Febrile status epilepticus
- Sudden reduction in antiepileptic medication
- Acute cerebral trauma
- Idiopathic epilepsy, i.e. cause unknown
- Bacterial meningitis
- Encephalopathy (including Reye's syndrome)
- Poisoning (BMJ 1997).

Aims of treatment:

- Maintain ABCD
- Stop fit
- Reduce risk of further fitting
- Treat cause
- Reduce risks associated with treatment.

Urgent investigations required:

- Glucose
- Sodium
- CT scan if suspect:
- Focal seizures
- Trauma
- Space-occupying lesion.

The treatment protocol for status epilepticus is set out in Figure 6.2. Thiopental is a general anaesthetic. It is particularly valuable in patients with neurological involvement because of its ability to acutely reduce ICP; it therefore has a cerebroprotective effect (Singer & Webb 1997).

It is an alkaline solution, which will cause irritation if it leaks into subcutaneous tissues – watch for signs of cannula extravasation.

By re-assessing the child after each step of the treatment protocol in Figure 6.2, or guidelines similar to it, the effects of treatment can be evaluated and the need for further intervention can be decided.

CERVICAL SPINE IMMOBILISATION

All children with serious trauma must be treated as though they have a cervical spine injury. It is only when adequate investigations have been performed and a neurosurgical or orthopaedic consultation obtained, if necessary, that the decision to remove cervical spine protection should be taken. In-line cervical stabilisation (Fig. 6.3) should be continued until a hard collar has been applied, and sandbags and tape or head blocks are in position as described below.

Two techniques are described. It is necessary to apply both to achieve adequate cervical spine control.

Once the collar is in place, the neck is largely obscured. Before placing the collar look for the following signs quickly and without moving the neck:

- Distended veins
- Tracheal deviation
- Wounds

Fig 6.2 Emergency treatment for convulsions (with permission from Advanced Life Support Group 2005)

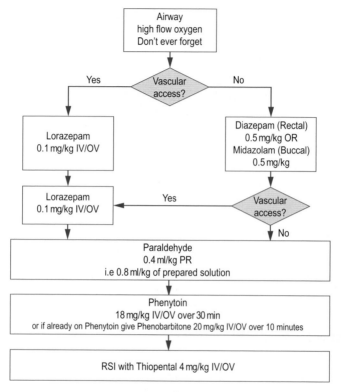

- Laryngeal crepitus
- Subcutaneous emphysema.

Application of a cervical collar

The key to a successful, effective collar application lies in selecting the correct size.

Minimum equipment

- Measuring device
- Range of paediatric hard collars

Fig 6.3 In-line cervical stabilisation (with permission from Advanced Life Support Group 2005)

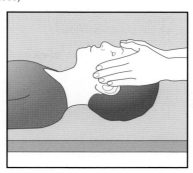

Method

1. Ensure that in-line cervical stabilisation is maintained throughout by a second person
2. Using the manufacturer's method, select a correctly sized collar
3. Fully unfold and assemble the collar
4. Taking care not to cause movement, pass the flat part of the collar behind the neck
5. Fold the shaped part of the collar round and place it under the child's chin
6. Fold the flat part of the collar with its integral joining device (usually Velcro tape) around until it meets the shaped part
7. Reassess the correct fit of the collar
8. If the fit is wrong, slip the flat part of the collar out from behind the neck, taking care not to cause movement. Select the correct size and recommence the procedure
9. If the fit is correct, secure the joining device
10. Ensure that in-line cervical stabilisation is maintained until head blocks and straps or sandbags and tape are in position.

Head blocks

Equipment

- Two head blocks
- Attachment system

Method

1. Ensure in-line cervical stabilisation is maintained by a second person throughout
2. Place a head block either side of the head
3. Apply the forehead strap and attach it securely
4. Apply lower strap across the chin piece of the hard collar and attach it securely
5. Apply tape across the chin piece of the hard collar and securely attach it to the long spinal board.

Exceptions

Two groups of children cause particular difficulty. The first (and most common) is the frightened, uncooperative child; the second is the child who is hypoxic and combative. In both cases, overzealous immobilisation of the head and neck may paradoxically increase cervical spine movement. This is because these children will fight to escape from any restraint. In such cases a hard collar should be applied, and no attempt should be made to immobilise the head with head blocks and straps or sandbags and tape.

Log-rolling

In order to minimise the chances of exacerbating unrecognised spinal cord injury, non-essential movements of the spine must be avoided until adequate examination and investigations have excluded it. If manoeuvres that might cause spinal movement are essential (e.g. during examination of the back in the course of the secondary survey) then log-rolling should be performed (Figs 6.4 and 6.5). The aim of log-rolling

Fig 6.4 Log-rolling a child (four-person technique) (with permission from Advanced Life Support Group 2005)

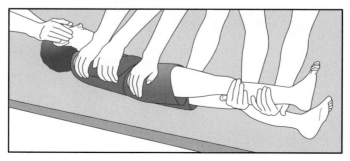

is to maintain the alignment of the spine during turning of the child. The basic requirements are an adequate number of carers and good control.

Method

1. Gather together enough staff to roll the child. In larger children four people will be required; three will be required in smaller children and infants
2. Place the staff as shown in Table 6.2
3. Ensure each member of staff knows what they are going to do, as shown in Table 6.3
4. Carry out essential manoeuvres as quickly as possible.

Fig 6.5 Log-rolling a small child or infant (three-person technique) (with permission from Advanced Life Support Group 2005)

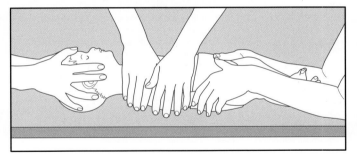

Table 6.2 Position of staff in log-rolling		
	Position of staff for:	
Staff member no.	**Smaller child and infant**	**Larger child**
1	Head	Head
2	Chest	Chest
3	Legs and pelvis	Legs
4		Pelvis

Source: with permission from Advanced Life Support Group 2005.

Table 6.3 Tasks of individual members of staff during log rolling

Staff member – position	Task
Head	Hold either side of the head (as for in-line cervical stabilisation) and maintain the orientation of the head with the body in all planes during turning **Control the log-roll by telling other staff when to roll and when to lay the child back on the trolley**
Chest	Reach over the child and carefully place both hands under the chest. When told to roll the child support the weight of the chest and maintain stability. Watch the movement of the head at all times and roll the chest at the same rate
Pelvis and legs	**This applies only to smaller children and infants. If it is not possible to control the pelvis and legs at the same time, get additional help immediately** Place one hand on either side of the pelvis over the iliac crests. Cradle the child's legs between the forearms. When told to roll the child, grip the pelvis and legs and move them together. Watch the movement of the head and chest at all times, and roll the pelvis and legs at the same rate
Pelvis	Place one hand over the pelvis on the iliac crest and the other under the top of the far leg. When told to roll the child watch the movement of the head and chest at all times and roll the pelvis at the same rate
Legs	Support the weight of the far leg by placing both hands under it. When told to roll the child watch the movement of the chest and pelvis and roll the leg at the same rate

Source: with permission from Advanced Life Support Group 2005.

SYNDROME OF INAPPROPRIATE ANTIDIURETIC HORMONE SECRETION

Syndrome of inappropriate antidiuretic hormone secretion (SIADH) can develop in any child who sustains injury to or compression of the pituitary or hypothalamus – this may occur as a result of:

- Head injury
- Intracranial haemorrhage
- Encephalopathies (including Guillain–Barré syndrome, meningitis and encephalitis)
- Hydrocephalus
- Raised ICP

- Neurosurgery
- Antidiuretic hormone (ADH)-secreting tumours.

ADH or arginine vasopressin is formed in the hypothalamus. It is transported to the posterior pituitary gland, where it is released in response to differences between extracellular and intracellular osmolality. ADH increases the permeability of the renal distal tubule and collecting ducts to water, so that less free water is excreted in the urine, reducing urine volume and increasing concentration. If ADH levels remain elevated, serum hypo-osmolality and hyponatraemia will develop.

Signs and symptoms

Urine volume is often reduced but the urine osmolality and sodium concentration will be high. If the SIADH continues, water intoxication and hyponatraemic seizures can result from the movement of water from the intravascular space into cerebral tissue.

Management

- Diagnosis is confirmed when patient responds to fluid restriction with correction of hyponatraemia
- Fluids usually restricted to 30–75% maintenance
- If profound hyponatraemia or signs of water intoxication are present (deterioration in level of consciousness or seizures), administration of hypertonic saline (3% sodium chloride) and a diuretic, e.g. furosemide, may be prescribed to increase serum sodium concentration and eliminate excess intravascular water
- Close monitoring of level of consciousness, fluid balance, daily weight, and blood and urine chemistries
- The underlying cause of the SIADH should be treated.

DIABETES INSIPIDUS

Central or neurogenic diabetes insipidus can be observed in children who sustain the following:

- Head injuries
- Central nervous system infections
- Intraventricular haemorrhages
- Neurosurgery.

Neurogenic diabetes insipidus results from decreased production of ADH. When ADH is not synthesised by the hypothalamus, circulating ADH levels are negligible. Renal collecting tubules therefore remain relatively impermeable to water, resulting in insufficient reabsorption. Large amounts of water are lost in urine. Intravascular volume is quickly depleted, and haemoconcentration produces hypernatraemia. The osmotic gradient causes fluid to shift from the intracellular to the intravascular space and that fluid is quickly lost from the circulation. Intravascular hypovolaemia stimulates aldosterone secretion, leading to the reabsorption of water and sodium from the proximal renal tubule. If the child's fluid intake is limited to intravenous therapy, and s/he is not able to drink freely, unrecognised diabetes insipidus can quickly produce hypovolaemia, hypernatraemia and serum hyperosmolality.

Signs and symptoms

- Polyuria – the excretion of large amounts of very dilute urine with low osmolality, low sodium concentration and very low specific gravity – important to detect this condition early because the critically ill child can become hypovolaemic and hypernatraemic very quickly
- Irritability, tachycardia, low CVP, weak peripheral pulses and hypotension, metabolic acidosis, prolonged capillary refill time
- In infant, anterior fontanelle depressed
- Reduced body weight.

Management

- Rapid replacement of urinary fluid and electrolyte losses and provision of ADH in the form of the drug DDAVP (vasopressin)
- Close monitoring of fluid balance, intravascular volume, systemic perfusion and electrolyte balance
- Positive response to vasopressin will be seen by decrease in urine volume to approximately 1 ml/kg/h, a rise in urine specific gravity to more than 1.010 and osmolality to 280–300 mmol/l (Hazinski 1992)
- By calculating fluid replacement on hourly urine output, it is easier to taper this in response to vasopressin.

GUILLAIN–BARRÉ SYNDROME

Guillain–Barré syndrome is the association of a preceding infection, progressive motor weakness and elevated CSF protein content. The preceding illness may be upper respiratory infection or viral illness. It most commonly occurs in children aged 4–10 years, although it can occur in any age group. The cause is unknown but appears to be related to an autoimmune or inflammatory processes that produce inflammation of nerves and nerve roots.

- The inflammation of the nerves and nerve roots involves the endodural and epidural blood vessels

- First the myelin becomes oedematous; demyelination develops, producing decreased speed and intensity of peripheral nerve conduction. Nerve degeneration may also occur.

Signs and symptoms

- Child may complain of tingling/numbness/pain in fingers and toes, and soon demonstrates weakness of the lower extremities and possible loss of deep tendon reflexes
- Over a period of several days or weeks, motor weakness ascends to include arms and possibly the cranial nerves. If the intercostal muscles are paralysed the child will require ventilatory assistance
- Glossopharyngeal and vagus nerve dysfunction may develop and produce impairment of the gag and swallow reflexes
- During the initial stages of the illness, autonomic instability may be evident, demonstrated by wide fluctuations in blood pressure, cardiac arrhythmias, diaphoresis (excessive sweating) and pupil dilation and constriction.

Recovery from Guillain–Barré syndrome usually begins approximately 4 weeks after the onset of symptoms. Although the majority of children make a complete recovery, a small number of affected patients die, some demonstrate significant neurological disorders and others may be prone to relapses.

Management

This is largely supportive, with weaning gradually taking place as the child recovers:

- Thorough and frequent neurological assessment, including limb strength and movement, and cranial nerve function
- Ventilation in order to protect airway as well as to assist child's own respiratory effort
- Careful monitoring of cardiovascular function, with treatment of arrhythmias and hypotension that result in a compromise of systemic perfusion
- Provision of adequate calorific intake (either enterally or parenterally)
- Plasmapheresis or intravenous Y globulin (Stack & Dobbs 2004)
- Physiotherapy and maintenance of skin integrity
- Psychological aspects of care (adapted from Hazinski 1992).

MYASTHENIA GRAVIS

Myasthenia gravis is a chronic disease (unless occurring in the neonatal period) marked by abnormal fatigability and weakness of selected muscles.

The degree of fatigue is so extreme that these muscles are temporarily paralysed. The muscles initially affected are those around the eyes, mouth and throat, resulting in drooping of the upper eyelids (ptosis), double vision and dysarthria (unclear speech). In extreme cases it can lead to respiratory failure. It is an autoimmune disease in which autoantibodies bind to cholinergic receptors on muscle cells, which impairs the ability of the transmitter acetylcholine to induce muscular contractions (adapted from Williams & Asquith 2000).

There are three types of myasthenia gravis seen in children:

- **Neonatal** Occurs in infants born to myasthenic mothers. It involves muscles associated with the distal cranial nerves, causing dysphonia, and dysphagia. It resolves spontaneously within the first 5 days of life
- **Congenital** Onset occurs within the first few days of life. Mothers of these infants rarely have myasthenia gravis but it may present in siblings. Respiratory failure is very unusual, but the infants will be poor feeders, and extraocular muscles will be affected.
- **Juvenile** May be present after the age of 2 years, but is most commonly present during adolescence. It first presents in the muscles supplied by the lower cranial nerves. This is the form of myasthenia gravis seen in adults (Willliams & Asquith 2000).

Management

- Diagnosis is made by titres for acetylcholine receptor antibodies, electromyogram (EMG) and a Tensilon test – Tensilon (edrophonium) is a short-acting anticholinergic drug given IV. The child will almost immediately show a dramatic, temporary increase in muscle strength
- Anticholinesterase drug therapy – commonly in the form of neostigmine or pyridostigmine
- Immunosuppression may reduce the production of acetylcholine receptor antibodies so corticosteroids may be used
- Plasmaphaeresis may give temporary remission as acetylcholine receptor antibodies are protein-bound
- Thymectomy may increase muscle strength as the thymus gland may increase the development of acetylcholine receptor antibodies; this may have long-term implications for the development of the immune system in children.

MENINGITIS

Meningitis is an acute inflammation of the meninges and CSF, which occurs more commonly in children than adults, particularly in children between 1 month and 5 years of age. It is most commonly caused by bacteria, although it can also be viral. In addition to *Neisseria meningitidis* and tuberculous meningitis, there is an age–related association with different causative organisms (Table 6.4).

Table 6.4	Causes of bacterial meningitis with age
0–2 months	Group B streptococci Enteric (*Escherichia coli, Klebsiella, Proteus, Listeria*
2–4 months	Group B streptococci *Streptococcus pneumoniae* *Haemophilus influenzae* type B Meningococcus
More than 4 months	*Streptococcus pneumoniae* Meningococcus *Haemophilus influenzae* type B (under 5s)

Source: with permission from Stack & Dobbs 2004.

Immunisation against *Haemophilus influenzae* type B (Hib vaccine), meningitis C and pneumococcus is now incorporated into the childhood immunisation schedule – see Chapter 13.

Signs and symptoms

- Difficult to assess in infants: extreme irritability, with high-pitched 'cerebral cry' or lethargy with vomiting and fever
- If intracranial pressure is high, anterior fontanelle may be full and tense
- Child may complain of headache and photophobia (extreme sensitivity to light)
- Neck stiffness
- Kernig's sign (pain associated with extension of the knee when the thighs are flexed)
- Brudzinski's sign (flexion of neck stimulates flexion at knees and hips).

The importance of early recognition of symptoms so that effective treatment can be commenced as soon as possible cannot be over-emphasised.

Management

Intubation and ventilation may be necessary to maintain a patent airway and to treat raised ICP

- If meningitis is suspected, while awaiting confirmation of diagnosis, the administration of IV antibiotics should commence – centres have their own protocols, but ceftriaxone and cefotaxime are the antibiotics of choice

- Full blood screen for analysis will be performed, including blood cultures
- Full neurological assessment in conjunction with holistic assessment
- Fluid restriction according to local policy
- Lumbar puncture to obtain CSF specimen may be performed **unless** the child is believed to have raised ICP, when it would be omitted
- Management of raised ICP if indicated, as discussed previously
- It is now common practice in many PICUs for children with meningitis to be nursed on an open unit, rather than in a cubicle, once the first dose of IV antibiotics has been given – refer to local infection control policy
- Once the causative agent has been identified, the appropriate antibiotics will be prescribed
- If the child shows signs of meningococcal sepsis, e.g. poor capillary refill time and toe–core gap, purpuric skin rash (small dark red spots (petechiae) caused by capillaries bleeding into the skin), deranged clotting and hypotension (late sign), that do not respond to boluses of fluid, multiorgan support including high-frequency oscillation, inotropes and renal replacement therapy may be required. For evidence based guidelines to manage sepsis see Chapter 10.

NB. Provision of prophylactic oral antibiotics to family members and others who have had recent, prolonged, close contact with the child, is common. Examples of these are ciprofloxacin or rifampicin. When rifampicin is administered, to avoid alarm, those taking it need to be informed that it turns bodily secretions, e.g. urine, red. If rifampicin is administered to women of childbearing age, it is important to inform them that this drug obliterates the action of the contraceptive pill.

Meningitis is a notifiable disease – the medical staff will have to therefore notify the public health inspector of the occurrence.

Viral meningitis may require only supportive care, as this form is usually much milder than bacterial meningitis.

THE CRANIAL NERVES (Table 6.5)

Many rhymes have been devised to help remember the cranial nerves. Here is an example:

On	Finn
Old	And (Acoustic – vestibulocochlear)
Olympus'	German
Towering	Viewed
Top	Some
A	Hops

Table 6.5 The cranial nerves

Cranial nerve	Function	Assessment
I Olfactory	Smell	Difficult to assess accurately in small children.
II Optic	Vision	Assess ability to see objects near and far, object moving into visual field from periphery and identifying colours.
III Oculomotor	Pupil constriction, movement of eye and eyelid	Pupils should constrict when light is applied to each; consensual constriction (constriction in response to light directed to other eye) should be observed; eye should follow moving object; eyelids should raise equally when eyes are open. Ptosis (drooping eyelid) and lateral downward deviation of eye with pupil dilatation + decreased response to light = oculomotor injury
IV Trochlear	Movement of eye (superior oblique muscle)	Assess ability of eyes to track object down through visual field – damage stops eyes moving downwards + medially. Diplopia (blurred or double vision) may be present
V Trigeminal	Sensation to most of face + movement of jaw	Cover eyes; sharp/soft to skin + assess sensation. Check clench + move jaw + chew
VI Abducens	Lateral movement of eye	Assess eye movement in socket tracking object – when object close to child, both eyes should track it + move together. Child may turn head towards weakened muscle to prevent diplopia
VII Facial	Motor innervation of face, sensation to anterior tongue + tears	Ask child to make faces (demonstrate) + assess symmetry of face. Tears should be produced when crying. Drops of sugar/salt on tongue – test taste

(continued on next page)

Table 6.5 The cranial nerves (continued)

Cranial nerve	Function	Assessment
VIII Vestibulocochlear (hearing)	Hearing + equilibrium	Clap hands – startle reflex in infants; blink reflex to sudden sound. NB. Cranial nerves III and IV must be intact for normal response to following: *Dolls eyes' manoeuvre (oculocephalic reflex)*: As child's head is turned, eyes should shift in sockets in direction **opposite** to head rotation; this constitutes the normal response *Cold water calorics (oculovestibular reflex)*: Normally, instillation of cold water into ear should produce lateral nystagmus (rapid involuntary movement of the eyes – up and down/side to side/rotating); not to be performed if child is conscious. These tests are typically performed as part of brain stem testing
IX Glossopharyngeal	Motor fibres to throat + voluntary muscles of swallowing + speech	Evaluate swallow, cough + gag (tests IX + X together). If possible assess clarity of speech
X Vagus	Sensory + motor impulses for pharynx	Test as above – particularly cough + gag
XI Spinal accessory	Major innervation of sternocleidomastoid + upper trapezius	Ask child to shrug shoulders and assess contraction of trapezius muscles; child to turn head as sternocleidomastoid muscle is palpated (long muscle in neck – serves to rotate head + flex neck)
XII Hypoglossal	Innervation of the tongue	Ask child to stick out tongue. Squeeze nose of infant – mouth should open + tip of tongue should rise in mouth

Source: adapted from McCance & Heuther 1992.

REFERENCES

Allen D 1993 Ventriculostomy. Surg Nurse July: 17–20

Advanced Life Support Group 2005 Advanced Paediatric Life Support: a practical approach, 4th edn. BMJ Publications, London

Birdsall C, Grief L 1990 How do you manage extraventricular drainage? Am J Nurs 90(11): 47–49

BMJ 1997 Advanced paediatric life support – the practical approach, 2nd edn. British Medical Journal, London

Center for Drug Administration and Research 2001 Pediatric exclusivity labeling changes. US Food and Drug Administration, Washington, DC. Available on line at: http://www.fda.gov/cder/pediatric/labelchange.htm. Accessed 5 September 2006

Chitnavis BP, Polkey CE 1998 ICP monitoring. Care Crit Ill 14(3): 80–84

Dee J, Park SY 2003 Lidocaine sprayed down the endotracheal tube attenuates the airway-circulatory reflexes by local anaesthesia during emergence and extubation. Anesth Analg 96: 293–297

Evans OB 1987 Manual of child neurology. Churchill Livingstone, New York

Feldman Z, Kanter M, Robertson C et al 1992 Effect of head elevation on intracranial pressure and cerebral blood flow in head injured patients. J Neurosurg 76: 207–211

Fisher MD 1997 Pediatric traumatic brain injury. Crit Care Nurs Q 20(1):36–51

Hazinski MF (ed) 1992 Nursing care of the critically ill child, 2nd edn. CV Mosby, St Louis, MO

Hsiang JK, Chesnut RM, Crisp CB et al 1994 Early, routine paralysis for intracranial pressure control in severe head injury: Is it necessary? Crit Care Med 22: 1471–1476

Johnston AJ, Steiner LA, Chatfield DA et al 2004 Effect of cerebral perfusion pressure augmentation with dopamine and norepinephrine on global and focal brain oxygenation after traumatic brain injury. Intens Care Med 30: 791–797

Kamat P, Vats A, Gross M, Checchia PA 2003 Use of hypertonic saline for the treatment of altered mental status associated with diabetic ketoacidosis. Pediatr Crit Care Med 4: 239–242

Khanna S, Davis D, Peterson B et al 2000 Use of hypertonic saline in the treatment of severe refractory posttraumatic intracranial hypertension in pediatric traumatic brain injury. Crit Care Med 28:1144

Lower J 2002 Facing neuro assessment fearlessly. Nursing 32(2): 58

McCance KL, Heuther S 1992 In: Hazinski MF (ed) Nursing care of the critically ill child, 2nd edn. CV Mosby, St Louis, MO

Piatt JH, Schiff SJ 1984 High dose barbiturate therapy in neurosurgery and intensive care. Neurosurgery 15: 427–444

Schinner K, Chisholm A, Grap M et al 1995 The effects of auditory stimuli on intracranial pressure and cerebral perfusion pressure in traumatic brain injury. J Neurosci Nurs 27: 348–354

Shann F, Henning R 2003 Paediatric Intensive Care Guidelines. Collective, Parkville, Victoria

Simpson D, Reilly P 1982 Paediatric coma scale. Lancet 2: 450

Singh NC (ed) 1997 Manual of pediatric critical care. WB Saunders, Philadelphia, PA

Singer M, Webb A 1997 Oxford handbook of critical care. Oxford University Press, Oxford

Shiozaki T, Sugimoto H, Taneda M et al 1998 Selection of severely head injured patients for mild hypothermia therapy. J Neurosurg 89: 206–211

Skippen P, Seear M, Poskitt K et al 1997 Effect of hyperventilation on regional cerebral blood flow in head-injured children. Crit Care Med 25: 1402–1409

Stack C, Dobbs P 2004 Essentials of paediatric intensive care. Greenwich Medical, London

Stringer T, Hasso AN, Thompson JR et al 1993 Hyperventilation-induced cerebral ischemia in patients with acute brain lesions: demonstration by xenon-enhanced CT. Am J Neuroradiol 14:475–484

Teasdale G, Jennett B 1974 Assessment of coma and impaired consciousness, a practical scale. Lancet 2: 81–84

Williams C, Asquith J (eds) 2000 Paediatric intensive care nursing. Churchill Livingstone, London

White JR, Farukhi Z, Bull C et al 2001 Predictors of outcome in severely head-injured children. Crit Care Med 29: 534–540

FURTHER READING

Foster C, Nadel S 2002 New therapies and vaccines for bacterial meningitis. Expert Opin Investig Drugs 11: 1051–1060

Society of Critical Care Medicine 2003 Guidelines for the acute medical management of severe traumatic brain injury in infants, children and adolescents. Crit Care Med Suppl 31: S417–S491

FLUIDS AND NUTRITION

7

When children are admitted to hospital, it is important to get an accurate weight, as fluids and medications are often based upon this. If the child presents in a critical condition then weighing the child would obviously be inappropriate; Table 7.1 therefore gives mean weights of babies and children on the 50th centile, which can be used as a guide, or an estimation can be calculated using the following formula.

GUIDELINES

Estimated body weight in a child aged 1–10 years of age:

$$\text{Weight (kg)} = (\text{Age in years} + 4) \times 2.$$

Table 7.2 is a guide to fluid requirements per 24 hours according to the age of the infant or child.

The daily fluid requirement chart serves as guidance only, as fluid requirements may be increased or decreased in certain circumstances:

- Increased fluids may be required in patients with a pyrexia, with burns requiring radiant heat, undergoing phototherapy or to replace lost volume

| Table 7.1 A guide to weight: mean weight of babies and children on 50th centile ||
Age	Mean weight (kg)
3 months	5.9
6 months	7.7
9 months	8.8
1 year	9.7
2 years	12
4 years	15.9
7.5 years	24
10.5 years	32.8
12.5 years	40
15.5 years	54.5

Source: adapted from Department of Health 1991. Crown copyright material is reproduced with the permission of the Controller of Her Majesty's Stationery Office.

Table 7.2 Daily fluid maintenance requirement in babies and children based on age and weight

Age/Weight	Fluid requirement
Newborn	60 ml/kg/24 h increasing by 10 ml/kg/d for 4 days
<10 kg	100 ml/kg/24 h
11–20 kg	1000 ml + 50 ml for each kg over 10 kg
21–30 kg	1500 ml + 25 ml for each kg over 20 kg up to a maximum of 2500 ml/day

Source: from Williams & Asquith 2000.

- Decreased fluids may be required in patients following cardiac surgery, or patients in renal or heart failure.

Table 7.3 Estimated average daily energy requirement by age

Age	Kilocalories/24 h
0–3 months	515–545
4–6 months	645–690
7–9 months	765–825
10–12 months	865–920
1–3 years	1165–1230
4–6 years	1545–1715
7–10 years	1740–1970
11–14 years	1845–2220
15–18 years	2110–2755

The lower end of the range refers to females and the upper end refers to males.
Source: from Department of Health 1991. Crown copyright material is reproduced with the permission of the Controller of Her Majesty's Stationery Office).

Table 7.3 shows recommended daily energy requirements for healthy infants and children, which will alter if the child becomes unwell or suffers trauma.

ENTERAL FEEDING

When infants or children are admitted to paediatric intensive care, enteral feeding is commenced whenever possible. Many units have developed practice guidelines to facilitate establishment of full enteral feeding within specified time limits. It may be necessary to give parenteral nutrition when feeding into the gastrointestinal tract is contraindicated or inadequate. Where possible, trophic enteral feeds should be administered alongside total parenteral nutrition (TPN) to maintain gut integrity. Consult paediatric dietitians wherever possible.

Nasogastric tube placement and use

Since many children in PICU are sedated and ventilated, nasogastric (NG) tubes are usually inserted to enable enteral feeding and the administration of oral medication. There is a small risk that the NG tube may be misplaced into the lungs on insertion or that the tube may become displaced out of the stomach at any stage. The National Patient Safety Agency (2005) reported 11 deaths in a 2-year period due to misplaced NG feeding tubes. It is therefore vital that staff consider the following before feeding via the NG tube:

- Correct and incorrect testing methods

Correct methods:
- Measuring the pH of aspirate using pH indicator strips is recommended (feeding can commence if pH is 5.5 or below)
- Radiography is recommended but should not be used routinely

Incorrect methods:
- 'Whoosh' test (auscultation of air insufflated through the feeding tube) – found to be an ineffective, unreliable method and where feeds were commenced there were some disastrous results (Metheny et al 1998)
- Testing acidity/alkalinity of aspirate using blue litmus paper. Blue litmus paper is not sensitive enough to distinguish between bronchial and gastric secretions (MHRA 2004)
- Interpreting absence of respiratory distress as an indicator of correct positioning. Small- and even large-bore NG tubes can enter the respiratory tract with few, if any, symptoms, particularly if the patient is unconscious (Metheny 2004, Torrington & Bowman 1981)
- Monitoring bubbling at the end of the tube is an unreliable method because the stomach also contains air and could falsely indicate respiratory placement (Metheny et al 1990)
- Observing the appearance of the NG aspirate is also unreliable as gastric and bronchial secretions can look similar (Hand et al 1984, Theodore et al 1984)

 None of the existing methods for testing the position of NG tubes is totally reliable.

- Carry out an individual risk assessment prior to administering anything via the NG tube, at least once daily during continuous feeds and following episodes of vomiting, retching or coughing
- Review and agree local action required

Fig. 7.1 Confirming the correct position of nasogastric feeding tubes in infants and children. Published by the National Patient Safety Agency in *Patient Safety Alert 05*, February 2005 (see www.npsa.nhs.uk/advice). The flowchart was developed to provide staff with a guide to minimise risk in placing nasogastric feeding tubes; however, staff should continue to make decisions based on individualised risk assessment appropriate to local circumstances, and to seek clinical and/or professional advice where necessary

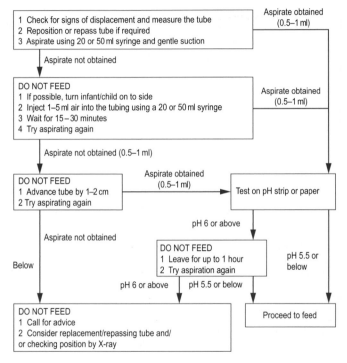

- Report misplaced incidents via local risk management reporting systems (National Patient Safety Agency 2005).

Figure 7.1 represents the correct procedure for commencing nasogastric feeds.

Nasojejunal feeding

In some situations it may be necessary to consider nasojejunal feeding where, for example, failure to absorb feeds as evidenced by gastric aspirates

---

Box 7.1   Principles of nasojejunal feeding

- Site nasojejunal tube according to local protocol
- Start feeds at recommended rate according to local protocol and feed for 4 hours
- After 4 hours, aspirate stomach contents:
  - If milky aspirates, nasojejunal tube not situated in the correct position so resite and start again
  - If no milky aspirates, increase rate of feeds every 4–6 hours until target volume is reached
- Monitor 4-hourly gastric aspirates for any sign of enteral feed
- Measure girth 12-hourly and, if girth increasing, discuss with medical colleagues regarding whether feeds should continue
- Monitor bowel movements, as bowels should open within 3 days of full enteral feeds with or without medication
- Transpyloric bolus feeds may cause diarrhoea, malabsorption and dumping syndrome – so continuous feeds are commonly recommended.

Source: adapted from protocols by R Meyer, Paediatric Research Dietitian, St Mary's Hospital, Paddington, London)

---

larger than the volume of feed instilled may indicate the failure of gastric emptying but not necessarily ileus (Box 7.1).

TYPES OF FEEDING AND PRODUCTS AVAILABLE

Breast feeding is the best form of nutrition for infants. Exclusive breast-feeding is recommended for the first 26 weeks of life (Department of Health 2003). Where possible, expressed or donated breast milk should be used as the preferred choice of feed for an infant from 0–6 months. There are, however, many products available to give a baby who for whatever reason cannot be breast-fed. Suitable products appropriate to age and weight for children in hospital who are unable to eat normally are discussed below.

Infant milks and children's feed (Royal College of Paediatrics and Child Health 2004)

Use of milk products and children's feeds

- Under 6 months of age use baby milk formula as preferred
- 6–12 months use formula as previous or follow-on formula
- Over 1 year use follow-on formula, full-fat cows' milk or standard child formula, e.g. Nutrini (1 kcal/ml), Nutrini Energy (1.5 kcal/ml).

Premature babies

Preterm babies with birthweight below 2 kg

- SMA low birthweight formula, Osterprem, Pre–Aptamatil, Nutriprem 1, PreNan.

Preterm babies above 2 kg until 6 months of age

- Premcare, Nutriprem 2.

Full-term babies

High energy for infants

These should only be used under dietetic supervision:

- Infatrini, SMA high energy formula.

Whey-based milks

These are the closest in composition to breast milk:

- SMA Gold, Cow & Gate Premium, Farleys First, Milupa Aptamil First.

Casein-based milks

- SMA White, Cow & Gate Plus, Farleys Second, Milupa Milumil.

Follow-on formulas

Only suitable from 6 months onwards:
- SMA Progress, Cow & Gate Step Up, Farleys Follow On, Milupa Aptamil Forward.

Soya milk

- Infasoy, Wysoy, Farleys soya formula, Prosobee, Isomil.

Concern has been raised over the use of soya formula in infants less than 6 months because of its phyto-oestrogen content. There is a potential risk that phyto-oestrogens could cause dysmenorrhoea in females and decreased fertility in males in later life. There are, however, three groups of infants in whom any potential risk of feeding soya formula is outweighed by the benefit:

- Infants with cow's milk protein allergy/intolerance who refuse extensively hydrolysed formulas
- Infants of vegan mothers
- Infants with galactosaemia.

Disaccharide/whole protein intolerance, e.g. cows milk protein intolerance

Extensively hydrolysed formulas are recommended as a first-line treatment in cows milk protein intolerance.

- Nutramigen, Prejomin, Peptite.

Elemental amino acid formula

Amino-acid-based infant formula can be used for cows milk protein allergy, multiple food intolerance, short bowel syndrome, protracted intractable diarrhoea.

- Neocate.

Infant low lactose formula

- Enfamil Lactofree, Galactomin 17, SMA LF.

Fructose-based and low-calcium infant formula

- Galactomin 19, Locasol.

Other products (for use in patients with chylothorax or liver disease)

- Monogen, MCT Pepdite, Caprilon.

Children's feeds

Standard whole protein feeds (1–6-year-olds/8–20 kg)

1 kcal/ml standard feeds:
- Nutrini, Frebini Original, PediaSure, Sondalis Junior.

1 kcal/ml standard feeds with fibre:
- Nutrini multifibre, Frebini Original Fibre, PediaSure Fibre.

High-energy whole protein feeds (1–6-year-olds/8–20 kg)

1.5 kcal/ml high-energy feeds:
- Nutrini Energy, Frebini Energy, PediaSure Plus.

1.5 kcal/ml high energy feeds with fibre:
- Nutrini Energy Multifibre, Frebini Energy Multifibre, PediaSure Plus Fibre.

Additional energy/protein supplements may be added to feeds under dietetic supervision. Supplements include:

- *Calories* – Duocal, Calogen, Maxijul
- *Protein* – Maxipro, Vitapro.

All formula milks in the UK are gluten-free (Shaw & Lawson 2001).

SPECIAL DIETS FOR SPECIAL KIDS

Infants and children with certain inborn errors of metabolism often have specific dietary requirements. General principles of dietary needs are highlighted; they are only intended as a guide to give nurses some ideas of general requirements and will not replace specialist advice from dietetic services.

Coeliac disease

- Coeliac disease is a malabsorption syndrome where the proximal intestinal mucosa lose their villous structure and the absorptive function becomes impaired
- It is precipitated by the ingestion of gluten in foods. Coeliac disease can result in severe symptoms such as steatorrhoea, abdominal discomfort and weight loss. This presentation, however, is quite rare and symptoms are usually less specific, e.g. iron-deficiency anaemia, fatigue or calcium deficiency
- A strict, lifelong gluten-free diet is required.

Cystic fibrosis

- Cystic fibrosis is a hereditary disorder with widespread dysfunction of exocrine glands, characterised by chronic pulmonary disease, pancreatic deficiency, abnormally high levels of electrolytes in the sweat and occasionally biliary cirrhosis
- Most patients will require pancreatic enzyme replacement therapy
- A high-protein, high-energy diet is required with added fat-soluble vitamins.

Diabetes mellitus

- Diabetes mellitus is a metabolic disorder where the pancreas becomes unable to maintain normal insulin production, causing hyperglycaemia, glycosuria and polyuria
- In children this is frequently controlled by a combination of diet and insulin
- A well balanced diet is required with minimal refined sugars, free fructose and an even distribution of carbohydrate throughout the day.

Inborn errors of metabolism

There are numerous disorders, which include disorders of amino acid metabolism, organic acidaemias and urea cycle defects. Details of each condition should be sought as only a brief outline will be given of a few disorders. Early discussion with a consultant who specialises in metabolic disorders is essential.

Phenylketonuria

- Phenylketonuria is a disorder of amino acid metabolism
- It is characterised by a deficiency of the liver enzyme phenylalanine hydroxylase, which is needed to break down the amino acid phenyl-alanine to tyrosine
- This disorder will be detected by the Guthrie test (a simple blood test taken once the infant is established on milk feeds and usually performed at around 1 week of age)
- Phenylalanine is essential for growth so, once the initially high level of phenylalanine has been reduced by a phenylalanine-free diet, it is gradually reintroduced at a low level
- A diet low in phenylalanine with a phenylalanine-free supplement of amino acids, vitamins and trace elements will be required for life.

Maple syrup urine disease

- Maple syrup urine disease is caused by a deficiency of branched chain 2-ketoacid dehydrogenase enzyme complex, which results in the accumulation of three branch chain amino acids – leucine, isoleucine and valine
- The infant presents in the first few days of life with encephalopathy, which may be mistaken for sepsis, and the characteristic urine that smells of maple syrup
- A low leucine diet is required with a branch-chain-free amino acid supplement, with vitamins and minerals
- If the child becomes unwell, all protein intake is stopped and an emergency regimen comprising the branch-chain-free supplement and additional calories is required. When these children become very sick, they may require haemofiltration to reduce the level of leucine.

Organic acidaemias

- There are several organic acidaemias, all due to different malfunctioning or absent enzymes resulting in a block of the breakdown of different amino acids
- The basic principles of dietary management include a low-protein diet and supplements of vitamins, minerals and trace elements; energy supplements are also required

- During periods of illness, the patient is at risk of developing metabolic acidosis due to accumulation of organic acids, so protein intake is usually withdrawn for a few days and an emergency diet, predominantly of a glucose polymer, e.g. Maxijul, or even total parenteral nutrition, is given (Shaw & Lawson 2001). In acute decompensation these children may have a rising level of lactate and may require haemofiltration
- Supplements of carnitine or other amino acid derivatives may be required. These patients may be on a low dose of metronidazole to reduce their gut flora, as propionic acid is formed in the gut.

Urea cycle defects

- Deficiencies of specific enzymes cause disorders in the urea cycle and lead to a build-up of ammonia in the blood and encephalopathy
- The infant or child may present with neurological abnormalities due to toxic levels of ammonia and acidosis and may require haemofiltration
- A low-protein diet is required to try to keep ammonia levels as low as possible, plus supplements of arginine (sodium benzoate, phenyl-acetate and citrulline may also be prescribed)
- In illness, the emergency regime of no protein with glucose polymer, Maxijul solution to supply calories may be imposed.

Glycogen storage diseases

Glucose-6-phosphatase deficiency

- This is an enzyme deficiency of glucose-6-phosphatase, which disrupts normal maintenance of plasma glucose levels
- It usually presents in infancy with hepatomegaly, hypoglycaemia and metabolic acidosis
- Frequent glucose/carbohydrate feeds and corn starch boluses are required to prevent hypoglycaemia
- In illness, an emergency regimen of glucose polymer, Maxijul solution is required to provide sufficient carbohydrate.

Galactosaemia

- Galactosaemia is an inborn error of galactose metabolism as a result of enzyme deficiency
- The majority of infants present in first week of life with jaundice, failure to thrive, vomiting, hepatomegaly and cataracts, as breast milk and most infant formulas contain galactose
- Treatment is a lifelong dairy-free diet. The infant formula of choice would be soya formula.

TOTAL PARENTERAL NUTRITION

Total parenteral nutrition consists of sterile solutions that are made up in pharmacy and are administered directly into the blood stream via a vein. The solutions:

- are made up of amino acids, carbohydrates and lipids
- should be protected from light to prevent the formation of free radicals
- should be stored in a fridge until used
- should be administered via a central line, especially if the glucose concentration is greater than 12.5%, and on a unique line saved for the sole use of TPN
- should be double-checked against the prescription before administration
- should be changed using aseptic precautions.

Patients on TPN should have daily weight, urine glucose and electrolytes, urea and electrolytes, full blood count, fluid balance and initially 6-hourly blood glucose tested. Every fortnight measure plasma chemistry for copper, manganese, selenium and zinc. (Adapted from Guy's, St Thomas', Kings College and Lewisham Hospitals 2005.)

On occasion it is necessary to make up solutions of dextrose that are not available as standard commercially prepared products (Table 7.4).

How to prepare 0.9% sodium chloride in 10% glucose

Remove 15 ml from a 500 ml bag of 10% glucose and discard. Draw up 15 ml of 30% sodium chloride and add to bag of 10% glucose and mix well.

How to prepare 3% solutions of sodium chloride

Remove 36 ml from a 500 ml bag of 0.9% sodium chloride and discard. Draw up 36 ml of 30% sodium chloride and add to the 0.9% sodium chloride bag.

- 4% and 0.18% dextrose saline solution contains 4 g of dextrose and 30 mmol of sodium and chloride per 100 ml

Table 7.4 How to prepare 12.5% and 15% glucose solutions		
Concentration required (%)	**Quantity of 50% glucose (ml)**	
12.5	31.25	Add to 468.75 ml of 10% glucose
15	62.5	Add to 437.5 ml of 10% glucose

- 5% dextrose contains 5 g dextrose/100 ml
- 10% dextrose contains 10 g dextrose/100 ml
- 50% dextrose contains 50 g dextrose/100 ml.

INSENSIBLE LOSS

This occurs mostly through the skin and the respiratory tract and accounts for approximately 30 ml/kg/24 h. However, fever will increase insensible loss by 12% per 1°C rise in temperature above 37.2°C (Shann 2003).

BURNS

See Chapter 10 for estimation of percentage burns and fluid replacement regimes.

REFERENCES

Department of Health 1991 Dietary reference values for food energy and nutrients for the United Kingdom. HMSO, London, p xix

Department of Health 2003 Maternal and infant nutrition. Department of Health, London. Available on line at www.dh.gov.uk/PolicyAndGuidance/HealthAndSocialCareTopics/MaternalAndInfantNutrition/fs/en (Accessed 19 September 2006)

Guy's, St Thomas', King's College and Lewisham Hospitals 2005 Paediatric formulary, 7th edn. Guy's, St Thomas', King's College and Lewisham Hospitals, London

Hand RW, Kempster M, Levy JH et al 1984 Inadvertent transbronchial insertion of narrowbore feeding tubes into the pleural space. JAMA 251: 2396–2397

Metheny NA, Aud MA, Ignatavicius DD 1998 Detection of improperly positioned feeding tubes. J Health Risk Manag 18(3): 37–48

Metheny N 1988 Measures to test placement of naso-gastric and naso-intestinal tubes: a review. Nurs Res 37: 324–329

Metheny N. 2004 Monitoring feeding tube placement – a literature review. Nutr Clin Pract 19: 487–495

Metheny N, Dettenmeier P, Hampton K et al 1990 Detection of inadvertent respiratory placement of small bore feeding tubes; a report of 10 cases. Heart Lung J Acute Crit Care 19: 631–638

MHRA 2004 MHRA MDA/2004/026 Enteral feeding tubes (nasogastric). Medicines and Healthcare Products Regulatory Agency, London

National Patient Safety Agency 2005 Reducing the harm caused by misplaced nasogastric feeding tubes. National Patient Safety Agency, London

Royal College of Paediatrics and Child Health 2004 Special foods for children. RCPCH Publications, London

Shann F 2003 Drug doses, 12th edn. Collective, Parkville, Victoria

Shaw V, Lawson M 2001 Clinical paediatric dietetics, 2nd edn. Blackwell, Oxford

Taylor S 1989 Preventing complications in enteral feeding. Prof Nurse 4: 247–249

Theodore AC, Frank JA, Ende J et al 1984 Errant placement of nasoenteric tubes. A hazard in obtunded patients. Chest 86: 931–933

Torrington KG, Bowman MA 1981 Fatal hydrothorax and empyema complicating a malpositioned nasogastric tube. Chest 79: 240–242

Williams C, Asquith J 2000 Paediatric intensive care nursing. Churchill Livingstone, London

FURTHER READING

McClaren DS, Burman D 1982 Textbook of paediatric nutrition, 2nd edn. Churchill Livingstone, Edinburgh

Taitz LS, Wardley B 1989 Handbook of child nutrition. Oxford University Press, Oxford

Useful websites

www.npsa.nhs.uk
www.nhsdirect.nhs.uk
www.breastfeeding.nhs.uk

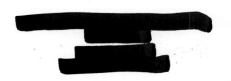

BLOOD AND ELECTROLYTES: NORMAL VALUES AND TRANSFUSION

8

This chapter highlights normal blood values, general information about blood products, storage and administration. Consult local policies and suppliers for further information. The normal ranges of blood values given are intended as a guide and may vary in different hospitals (Tables 8.1–8.4).

NORMAL VALUES: FULL BLOOD COUNT

Table 8.1 Full blood count for normal infants and children

Age	Units	Newborn full-term	Up to 6 months	2–6 years	6–12 years
Red blood cells (RBC)	$\times 10^{12}$/l	6.0 ± 1.0	3.8 ± 0.8	4.6 ± 0.7	4.6 ± 0.6
Haemoglobin (Hb)	g/dl	16.5 ± 3.0	11.5 ± 2.0	12.5 ± 1.5	13.5 ± 2.0
Packed cell volume (PCV)	l/l	0.54 ± 0.10	0.35 ± 0.07	0.37 ± 0.03	0.40 ± 0.05
Mean corpuscular volume (MCV)	fl	110 ± 10	91 ± 17	81 ± 6	86 ± 8
Mean corpuscular haemoglobin (MCH)	pg	34 ± 3	30 ± 5	27 ± 3	29 ± 4
Platelets	$\times 10^9$/l	150–400	150–400	150–400	150–400
White blood count (WBC)	$\times 10^9$/l	18 ± 8	12 ± 6	10 ± 5	9 ± 4
Neutrophils	$\times 10^9$/l	5.0–13.0	1.5–9.0	1.5–8.0	2.0–8.0
Lymphocytes	$\times 10^9$/l	3.0–10.0	4.0–10.0	6.0–9.0	1.0–5.0
Monocytes	$\times 10^9$/l	0.7–1.5	0.1–1.0	0.1–1.0	0.1–1.0
Eosinophils	$\times 10^9$/l	0.2–1.0	0.2–1.0	0.2–1.0	0.1–1.0
Reticulocytes	$\times 10^9$/l	200–500	40–100	20–200	20–200

Source: from Dacie & Lewis 1997.

CLOTTING VALUES

Table 8.2   Clotting values

	Abbreviation	Value	Standard unit
Prothrombin time	PT	11–16	Seconds
International normalised ratio	INR	0.8–1.1	Ratio
Activated prothrombin time	APTT	0.8–1.2	Ratio
Fibrinogen		2.02–4.24	g/l

UREA AND ELECTROLYTES

Table 8.3   Urea and electrolytes

	Value	Standard units
Sodium	135–145	mmol/l
Potassium	3.5–5.0	mmol/l
Chloride	98–107	mmol/l
Bicarbonate	22–32	mmol/l
Anion gap	7–17	mmol/l
Urea	2.5–7.5	mmol/l
Creatinine	40–90	μmol/l
Calcium	2.19–2.51	mmol/l
Alb. corrected calcium	2.19–2.51	mmol/l
Magnesium	0.65–0.95	mmol/l
Phosphate	1.2–1.8	mmol/l
Total protein	62–81	g/l
Albumin	37–56	g/l
Alkaline phosphatase	145–320	U/l
Total bilirubin	0–22	μmol/l
Alanine transaminase	0–55	U/l
Aspartate transaminase	0–35	U/l
Gamma glutamyl transpeptidase	8–78	U/l
C reactive protein	<7	mg/l

NORMAL BLOOD VOLUMES

- Preterm babies approximately 100 ml/kg
- Infants approximately 80 ml/kg
- Children approximately 70 ml/kg.

TRANSFUSION COMPATIBILITY

Blood should be cross-matched before the patient is transfused wherever possible but in emergency situations blood group O Rh D negative is sometimes used. For neonates in an emergency situation, red cells are suspended in citrate, phosphate, glucose (anticoagulant) and will be sickle Hb-positive, cytomegalovirus (CMV)-positive and Kell antigen-positive.

Table 8.4 Transfusion compatibility for ABO group and Rhesus factor

	Whole blood	Platelets	Fresh frozen plasma	Cryoprecipitate	Human albumin solution
Blood group O	O	O	Any	O	Any
Blood group A	A or O	A or O	A or AB	A	Any
Blood group B	B or O	B or O	B or AB	A*	Any
Blood group AB	Any	Any	AB	A*	Any
Special giving set/filter required	Blood giving set	Platelet giving set	Blood giving set	Blood or platelet giving set	No

* Many transfusion centres only produce group O or A cryoprecipitate.
Source: adapted with permission from Shann 2003.

TRANSFUSION COMPONENTS

Red cells, red cells with additives

Whole blood or packed cells are transfused where major blood loss has occurred, for haemoglobinopathies and in patients with severe anaemias.

Once plasma has been removed from whole blood, additives are used to re-suspend red cells and these are designed to maintain the red cells in optimum condition during storage.

- **Red cells CPDA** = added citrate, phosphate, dextrose and adenine
- **Red cells SAGM** = added sodium chloride, adenine, glucose and mannitol.

Component volumes to be transfused to neonates and children

Red cell concentrates

Top up transfusion: Desired Hb (g/dl) − actual Hb × weight (kg) × 4, or 15 ml/kg.

The recommended rate of transfusion of red cell products is 5 ml/kg/h (British Committee for Standards in Haematology Transfusion Taskforce 2004).

Fresh frozen plasma

Fresh frozen plasma (FFP) is often used following cardiopulmonary bypass to help correct prolonged clotting times and improve haemostasis, or may be used where there is evidence of microvascular bleeding and abnormal coagulation.

This occasionally causes severe anaphylactic reactions, especially if infused rapidly.

Dosage is dependent on the clinical condition of the patient, but 10–20 ml/kg may be used.

FFP does not transmit CMV and does not need to be irradiated.

FFP for patients born after 1 January 1996 in the UK is now pooled and treated with methylene blue for viral inactivation (as those children have not been exposed to bovine spongiform encephalopathy (BSE) in the foodchain).

Indications for use:
- In bleeding or unstable patient where INR or APTT > 1.5
- Prior to invasive procedure if INR or APTT > 1.5 (consider vitamin K first)
- To treat thrombotic thrombocytopenia purpura
- Reversal of warfarin excess according to local protocol (prothrombin complex concentrate may be preferable).

Half-life: around 4 days in the circulation.

Platelets

Platelets may be given where severe microvascular bleeding occurs, e.g. in disseminated intravascular coagulation (DIC).

These should preferably be ABO- and Rh D-compatible as a transfusion could contain enough volume of plasma from a single donor to cause a risk of haemolysis if the donor has potent cell antibodies.

Carefully look at the pooled platelets before giving as they are stored at room temperature and therefore prone to bacterial contamination. If discoloured or visible clumping is observed, **do not give** – refer back to the lab that produced them. Platelet infusion occasionally results in severe anaphylactic reaction, especially if infused too quickly.

Indications

- Patients with thrombocytopenia secondary to marrow failure
  - In a stable patient maintain platelets above $10 \times 10^9/l$
  - In a patient with sepsis, bleeding or who is ventilated, target platelet threshold of $50 \times 10^9/l$

- To cover an invasive procedure, e.g. central line insertion, platelet count should be $50 \times 10^9/l$
- For surgery/ invasive procedures in critical sites, e.g. CNS, aim for platelet count of $100 \times 10^9/l$
- Patients with thrombocytopenia secondary to peripheral consumption (not immune thrombocytopenia purpura)
  - Stable patients not on anticoagulants, not bleeding, not in ITU, keep platelets above $10 \times 10^9/l$
  - Unstable patients who are receiving anticoagulants, critically ill or bleeding, aim for platelets of $50 \times 10^9/l$
  - Patients with uncontrolled bleeding or haemorrhage in critical site, maintain platelets above $100 \times 10^9/l$

 Platelet transfusion is contra-indicated in patients with thrombotic thrombocytopenia purpura and heparin induced thrombocytopenia.

 Patients with immune thrombocytopenia purpura (ITP) should only be given platelets under the guidance of a haematologist.

Guidelines for platelet transfusion in newborn infants:
- The risk of bleeding in newborn infants is increased when the platelet count $< 100 \times 10^9/l$.
- Platelet transfusion thresholds in neonates are as follows:
  - $20 \times 10^9/l$ in otherwise well infants
  - $30 \times 10^9/l$ in infants with sepsis or abnormal coagulation
  - $50 \times 10^9/l$ in the presence of bleeding
  - $100 \times 10^9/l$ in the presence of intracranial or other life-threatening bleeding.

Half-life: 5 days in circulation.

Dose: dependent on clinical condition, usually 10–20 ml/kg

Cryoprecipitate

Cryoprecipitate will be given to increase the fibrinogen level, e.g. in a patient who has developed DIC.

This is obtained by allowing the frozen plasma from a single donation to thaw at 4°C and removing the supernatant. It is rich in factor VIII, von Willebrand's factor and fibrinogen. Cryoprecipitate has not been shown to transmit CMV and does not need irradiating.

This occasionally can cause severe anaphylactic reactions if infused rapidly.

Indications: use in bleeding patient where fibrinogen is low (<0.8–1.5 g/dl)

Dose: usually 5–10 ml/kg.

Gelofusine

This is a sterile modified fluid gelatin in saline, a colloidal plasma volume substitute. Gelofusine can increase blood volume, cardiac output, stroke volume, blood pressure, urine output and oxygen delivery.

Half-life: around 4 h – the majority of the dose is eliminated by renal excretion within 24 h.

4.5% human albumin solution

This is used for volume replacement of plasma, e.g. in clinical management of hypovolaemic shock or burns. The only benefit over other colloidal solutions is a longer half-life but it is much more expensive.

Half-life: around 19 days in a healthy adult (no information regarding half-life in children).

The use of human albumin solution is currently under review. Consult local policy for use.

Box 8.1 Clinical guidelines for the use of irradiated blood products

Cellular blood products such as red cells, platelets and granulocytes (neutrophils) or buffy coat (white cell) preparations are irradiated in certain situations to prevent the occurrence of transfusion related graft versus host disease (TA-GVHD), a fatal complication of transfusion, which is most likely to occur in the immunocompromised patient.

Irradiated blood products should be ordered in the following situations:

- All blood for intrauterine transfusions
- All subsequent transfusions for babies who have received intrauterine transfusions
- All blood for exchange transfusions in neonates
- All patients with suspected congenital immunodeficiency, with the exception of chronic mucocutaneous candidiasis
- All HLA-matched products or products donated by family members
- All patients with Hodgkin's disease
- Patients who have received purine analogue therapy (fludarabine, 2-CDA or deoxycoformycin)
- All granulocyte or buffy coat preparations
- All patients who have undergone or are within 6 weeks of undergoing autologous or allogenic bone marrow transplantation
- All patients within 1 week of bone marrow or peripheral stem cell harvest.

Source: adapted by Dr C Harrison from British Committee for Standards in Haematology Transfusion Taskforce 2004.

Box 8.2 Clinical guidelines for the use of cytomegalovirus-negative products

CMV-negative products are given to patients who are vulnerable to transfusion-acquired CMV infection.

CMV-negative products should be requested for:

- All components for children under 1 year
- All intrauterine transfusions
- All HIV-positive patients
- All CMV-negative patients who are potential candidates for stem cell or solid organ transplant
- All CMV-negative patients who are within 6 months of an autologous marrow transplant.

Please adhere to local policies and guidelines.

Source: adapted by Dr C Harrison from British Committee for Standards in Haematology Transfusion Taskforce 2004.

Table 8.5 Blood components – storage and administration

	Storage temperature (°C)	Shelf life	Longest time from leaving storage to finishing transfusion
Red cells/whole blood	2–6	35 d	5 h
Platelets	20–24 on agitator rack	5 d	Consult supplier
Fresh frozen plasma	−30	1 year frozen	4 h after thawing
Cryoprecipitate	−30	1 year frozen	4 h after thawing

Source: adapted from McClelland 1996. Crown copyright material is reproduced with the permission of the Controller of Her Majesty's Stationery Office.

Red cell products

Added chemicals are used to re–suspend packed red cells after plasma has been removed (Table 8.5). They are designed to maintain the cells in good condition during storage. Do not add any drugs or additives to blood products received (e.g. calcium can cause citrated blood to clot, 5% dextrose can lyse red cells).

Blood components

It is important to follow local policies and protocols when ordering and administering blood products. Table 8.5 provides guidelines regarding storage, shelf life and recommended transfusion times.

Blood filters

All blood products should be given through an appropriate giving set with an integral filter. Whole blood, packed cells, fresh frozen plasma and cryoprecipitate can be given through a blood giving set while platelets require a special giving set.

Blood warmers

If cold blood is infused too quickly, cardiac arrest can occur. Blood warmers should have a visible thermometer and audible alarm. If red cells and plasma are exposed to temperatures in excess of 40°C, severe transfusion reactions can occur. Blood should not be warmed by any other method.

Transfusion

During the transfusion of the blood product, observe the patient for signs of incompatibility or adverse reaction, e.g. fever, flushing, vomiting, urticaria, diarrhoea, itching, headache, rigors, haemoglobinuria, severe backache, pain at transfusion site, collapse, circulatory failure. If any of these signs are observed, stop the transfusion, inform the doctor and keep the intravenous line open with normal saline. Acute haemolytic transfusion reactions can be fatal and the patient may require adrenaline (epinephrine) and chlorphenamine (chlorpheniramine).

Special requirements – premature babies

In preterm babies a formal cross-match may be considered unnecessary in the first 4 months of life if there are no passively acquired maternal antibodies. CMV-negative, blood group O, Rhesus-negative blood with low anti-A and anti-B titres is usually provided in neonatal units and is suitable for neonates of any ABO and Rhesus D group.

Red cells must be transfused through a 20 µm filter to remove microaggregates.

PLATELET DISORDERS

Thrombocytopenia is caused by a reduction in platelet production or excessive peripheral destruction. Common causes of thrombocytopenia found in children are listed in Box 8.3.

DIC is discussed as this may be seen in children presenting to paediatric intensive care or may develop, e.g. secondary to meningococcal disease.

Disseminated intravascular coagulation

DIC refers to a spectrum of haemostatic disorders characterised by a reduction in factor V, factor VIII, fibrinogen and platelets. Widespread

---

Box 8.3 Common causes of thrombocytopenia in infants and children

Placental factors
- Infarction angiomas
- Lupus anticoagulants

Maternal factors
- Immune thrombocytopenia
- Intrauterine infections, e.g. toxoplasmosis, rubella, CMV, herpes simplex
- Pre-eclampsia
- Drugs

Infant factors
- Disseminated intravascular coagulation
- Primary microangiopathic haemolytic anaemias, e.g. haemolytic–uraemic syndrome
- Giant haemangioma syndrome
- Hypercoagulable states
- Birth asphyxia
- Cyanotic congenital heart disease
- Respiratory distress syndrome
- Necrotising enterocolitis
- Bacterial infection
- Rhesus haemolytic disease
- Anticoagulant deficiency
- Heparin-induced thrombocytopenia
- Rare bone marrow diseases

Source: adapted with permission from Lilleyman et al 2000.

---

intravascular coagulation occurs, with secondary activation of fibrinolysis caused by excessive production of thrombin.

Clinical presentation: A patient with DIC may have no obvious signs of bleeding, merely abnormal clotting results or may present acutely ill, in shock, tachycardic, hypotensive, bleeding from venepuncture sites, nose, mouth as well as having signs of pulmonary and cerebral bleeds. Tissue necrosis may occur as a result of thrombus in peripheral veins.

Patients with DIC may have:

- decreased platelets
- low fibrinogen
- increased fibrin degradation product
- extended prothrombin time
- extended partial thromboplastin time
- abnormal factors V and VIII.

Treatment:
- Treat primary disease or precipitant
- Give blood products as indicated.

Box 8.4 Common causes of disseminated intravascular coagulation

- Sepsis
- Haemolytic transfusion reactions
- Burns
- Fresh water drowning
- Snake bites

The role of heparin is controversial and may be indicated in a predominantly thrombotic DIC. The indications for its use depend on individual unit policy. Activated protein C or antithrombin 111 are more frequently used.

REFERENCES

British Committee for Standards in Haematology Transfusion Taskforce 2004 Transfusion guidelines for neonates and older children. Br J Haematol 124: 433–453
Dacie JV, Lewis SM 1997 Practical haematology, 8th edn. Churchill Livingstone, Edinburgh
Lilleyman J, Hann I, Blanchette V 2000 Pediatric hematology, 2nd edn. Churchill Livingstone, Edinburgh
McClelland B (ed) 1996 Handbook of transfusion medicine, 2nd edn. HMSO, London
Shann F 2003 Drug doses, 12th edn. Collective, Parkville, Victoria

DRUGS – INOTROPES, VASODILATORS, SEDATIVES, ANALGESICS AND MUSCLE RELAXANTS

9

This chapter is intended for use as a quick reference guide and it is not designed to replace the British National Formulary, the Association of the British Pharmaceutical Industry Data Sheet Compendium, paediatric formularies or any other sources of specialist information about drug use in children.

Great care has been taken to ensure that the dosages given are correct at the time of writing but dose schedules do change and relevant information sources should be used to check doses when necessary.

NB. Many drugs discussed in this chapter are unlicensed for use in children.

RESUSCITATION DRUGS

Drugs that may be used during resuscitation are outlined in Table 9.1. See also Chapter 1.

Guidance regarding the indications for each of these drugs should be sought before use.

Adrenaline (epinephrine) 0.1 ml of 1:1000 is no longer recommended so subsequent doses should remain as 0.1 ml of 1:10 000. Anecdotal cases where larger doses of adrenaline have led to a return of spontaneous circulation have been reported, indicating that patient responses to adrenaline are variable and that larger doses are occasionally used.

Table 9.1 Resuscitation drugs

Drug	Use	Intravenous dose
Atropine sulphate	Sinus bradycardia	20 μg/kg*
Calcium chloride 10%	Acute hypotension	0.1–0.2 ml/kg
Adrenaline (epinephrine)	Cardiac arrest:	0.1 ml/kg of 1:10 000
Sodium bicarbonate 8.4%	Correction of metabolic acidosis	1 ml/kg for infants and children
Sodium bicarbonate 4.2%	Correction of metabolic acidosis	2 ml/kg for neonates
Naloxone	Reversal of opioid-induced respiratory depression	10 μg/kg

* The **minimum** dose of atropine sulphate that should be given is 100 μg to produce vagolytic effects and avoid paradoxical bradycardia (American Heart Association 1997).

See Chapter 1 for details of drugs that can be given via the endo-tracheal route.

DRUGS FOR INTUBATION

To reduce the risk of damaging the upper airway during intubation, infants and children should be sedated and paralysed prior to the procedure. The sedatives and neuromuscular blocking drugs commonly used as premedication for intubation are outlined in Table 9.2. Comprehensive

Table 9.2 Drugs for intubation

Drug	Use	Dose (IV)	Comments
Atracurium	Non-depolarising neuromuscular blocking agent	Initially 300–600 µg/kg	Often drug of choice in patients with renal or hepatic impairment Can cause histamine release so avoid in asthma Short to intermediate duration of action
Pancuronium	Non-depolarising neuromuscular blocking agent	30–40 µg/kg in neonates 60–100 µg/kg in children	Long duration of action (60–120 min) No histamine release but can cause tachycardia and hypertension Use with caution in severe renal and liver failure as duration is prolonged
Rocuronium	Non-depolarising neuromuscular blocking agent	0.6 mg/kg stat	Duration of action: infants 40 min, children 30 min Advantages over atracurium or vecuronium, include rapid onset of action within 60 s, cardiovascular stability, no drug accumulation or histamine release Duration prolonged in liver failure but do not adjust intubation dose In myasthenia gravis, use smaller dose of 0.2 mg/kg (NB. long duration of action) NB. In emergencies, rocuronium can be given via the IM route in deltoid muscle: dose 1 mg/kg <1 year or 2 mg/kg >1 year, but onset of action takes 4 min (Fisher 1999)
Suxamethonium	Depolarising neuromuscular blocking agent	2 mg/kg in neonates and infants	Very rapid onset of action (1 min), but very short duration of action (4–6 min)

Drug	Use	Dose (IV)	Comments
		1–2 mg/kg in children Maximum dose 2.5 mg/kg	May cause bradycardia in children, especially following a second dose Not recommended in liver disease, burns or patients with Duchenne muscular dystrophy Can cause profound hyperkalaemia, especially in burns, trauma and patients with renal failure
Ketamine	General anaesthetic agent	1–2 mg/kg	Contraindicated in hypertension. Risk of hallucinations is higher in older children and teenagers Coadministration of a benzodiazepine reduces the risk of hallucinations
Fentanyl	Opiate analgesic	1–5 μg/kg	Short-acting but potentially cumulative. At higher doses, risk of rigid chest syndrome
Morphine	Opioid sedative and analgesic	50–100 μg/kg in neonates 100–200 μg/kg in infants and children	Neonates and infants show increased susceptibility to respiratory depression
Thiopentone	Used for induction of anaesthesia	2 mg/kg in neonates 4–6 mg/kg in >1 month	Acutely reduces intracranial pressure and reduces cerebral metabolism, so may be drug of choice in patients with head injury (Singer & Webb 1997)

Source: information collated from Guy's, St Thomas', King's College and University Lewisham Hospitals 2005.

prescribing information should be consulted before prescribing or administering these drugs.

QUICK REFERENCE GUIDE FOR CALCULATING INFUSIONS

Many units use standard infusion calculations. Table 9.3 shows some of these 'rules of thumb' for frequently used drugs in paediatric intensive care.

These are not designed to replace infusion checking calculations which must always be performed when making up infusions. All infusions are made up to 50 ml.

Table 9.3 Standard preparation for common intravenous drug infusions

Drug	Quantity	Diluent up to 50 ml	Dose if run at 1 ml/h	Administration Central	Peripheral
Adrenaline (epinephrine)	0.3 mg × weight (kg)	0.9% saline or 5% glucose	0.1 µg/kg/min	✓	
Aminophylline	50 mg × weight (kg)	0.9% saline or 5% glucose	1 mg/kg/h	✓	✓
Clonidine	25 µg × weight (kg)	0.9% saline or 5% glucose	0.5 µg/kg/h	✓	✓
Dinoprostone (prostaglandin E_2)	30 µg × weight (kg)	0.9% saline or 5% glucose	10 ng/kg/min	✓	✓
Dobutamine	30 mg × weight (kg)	0.9% saline or 5% glucose	10 µg/kg/min	✓	
Dopamine	30 mg × weight (kg)	0.9% saline or 5% glucose	10 µg/kg/min	✓	
Dopamine	3 mg × weight (kg)	0.9% saline or 5% glucose	1 µg/kg/min		✓
Furosemide	10 mg × weight (kg)	0.9% saline	200 µg/kg/h	✓	✓
Glyceryl trinitrate	3 mg × weight (kg)	0.9% saline or 5% glucose	1 µg/kg/min	✓	✓
Midazolam	3 mg × weight (kg)	0.9% saline or 5% glucose	1 µg/kg/min	✓	✓
Milrinone	1.5 mg × weight (kg)	0.9% saline or 5% glucose	0.5 µg/kg/min	✓	✓
Morphine	1 mg × weight (kg)	0.9% saline or 5% glucose	20 µg/kg/h	✓	✓
Noradrenaline (norepinephrine)	0.3 mg × weight (kg)	0.9% saline or 5% glucose	0.1 µg/kg/min	✓	
Salbutamol	3 mg × weight (kg) (max 25 mg/50 ml)	0.9% saline or 5% glucose	1 µg/kg/min	✓	✓
Sodium nitroprusside*	3 mg × weight (kg) (max 50 mg/50 ml)	0.9% saline or 5% glucose	1 µg/kg/min	✓	✓
Vecuronium	5 mg × weight (kg)	0.9% saline or 5% glucose	100 µg/kg/h	✓	✓

* Sodium nitroprusside when made up must be protected from light and if available an amber giving set can be used.
Source: information collated from Guy's, St Thomas', King's College and University Lewisham Hospitals 2005.

Checking the infusion dose from the syringe concentration:

- Use the prescribed drug dose, i.e. the total amount in the 50 ml syringe × 1000 to give amount in nanograms or micrograms if the units differ from the prescription
- Divide this by 50 to give the amount per millilitre
- Divide by the weight in kilograms to give amount per kilogram per millilitre
- (Divide this figure by 60 if the infusion is calculated dose/kg/min).

INOTROPIC AND CHRONOTROPIC DRUGS

An inotrope is a drug that increases the force of cardiac muscular contraction.

A chronotrope is a drug that alters the heart rate, i.e. the rate of contraction of the heart.

Inotropic and chronotropic drugs are used in clinical practice. The effects produced by inotropic and chronotropic drugs are largely dependent upon the receptor sites activated and the doses administered. Table 9.4 outlines the receptor selectivity and pharmacological effects produced by commonly used agents.

DRUGS COMMONLY USED AS INTRAVENOUS INFUSIONS

Adenosine

Pharmacology: Adenosine is an endogenous nucleoside acting on coronary perfusion and myocardial conduction. It inhibits noradrenaline (norepinephrine) release from nerve endings, causes vasodilation and has important antiarrhythmic properties. Adenosine has diverse physiological functions mediated by receptors A_1, A_{2A}, A_{2B} and A_3. Actions mediated by A_1 receptors include slowing the heart rate and blocking atrioventricular nodal conduction, reduction of atrial contractility, attenuation of the stimulatory actions of catecholamine release on the heart. It also produces constriction of bronchial smooth muscle receptors by A_1 stimulation in asthmatics.

Adenosine is a rapidly acting drug with a half-life of less than 10 seconds.

Indications: Rapid reversion to sinus rhythm of supraventricular tachycardias, or as an aid to diagnosis of broad or narrow complex supraventricular tachycardias

Monitoring: Continuous ECG monitoring, blood pressure

Side effects: Transient facial flush, chest pain, dyspnoea, bronchospasm, choking sensation, severe bradycardia

Table 9.4 The pharmacological effect and receptor selectivity of various inotropic and chronotropic drugs

	Receptor selectivity			Pharmacological effect				
	α	β₁	β₂	Peripheral vascular vasodilation	Peripheral vascular vasoconstriction	Inotropic	Chronotropic
Dobutamine	+	+++	++	++	−	+++	+
Dopamine 0.5–2 μg/kg/min	−	−	−	− (renal and splanchnic dilatation)	−	−	−
Dopamine 2–5 μg/kg/min	−	+	−	+ (renal and splanchnic dilatation)	+	+	+
Dopamine > 5 μg/kg/min	+	++	−	− (renal and splanchnic dilatation)	++	++	++
Enoximone	−	−	−	+	−	+++	++
Epinephrine	+	+++	++	++	−	+++	++
Isoprenaline	−	++++	+++	+++	−	+++	+++
Noradrenaline (norepinephrine)	++++	++	−	−	++++	+	+

Source: with permission from Young & Koda-Kimble 1995.

Dosage and administration: Initial dose 100 μg/kg, then increase dose to 200 μg/kg, then 300 μg/kg if conversion to normal sinus rhythm has not been achieved. The maximum total dose should be 500 μg/kg (300 μg/kg under one month) (Advanced Life Support Group 2006). Fast IV bolus injection over less than 2 seconds followed by 5–10 ml rapid bolus of 0.9% sodium chloride. Give centrally if access available or into a large peripheral vein as it is rapidly metabolised in the peripheral circulation and administration is painful.

Contraindications
- Adenosine may not be drug of choice in asthmatics as it can cause bronchospasm
- It is contraindicated in heart block
- If patient is on concurrent dipyridamole, the initial dose of adenosine should be quartered. The reason for this is not fully understood, but dipyridamole increases plasma levels of endogenous adenosine by inhibiting its uptake into cells (German et al 1989)

Adrenaline (epinephrine)

Pharmacology: Adrenaline is a potent agonist of α-, β_1- and β_2-adrenoreceptors and has very low affinity for dopamine receptors. The effects it produces are dependent upon this receptor sensitivity. β_1-receptor stimulation produces positive inotropy, increasing cardiac output and systolic blood pressure. β_2-receptor stimulation produces skeletal muscle vasodilation, which results in reduced peripheral vascular resistance and often a fall in diastolic blood pressure. At higher doses, α_1-receptor stimulation becomes increasingly significant and produces peripheral vasoconstriction, resulting in increases in peripheral resistance and diastolic blood pressure.

Indications: Inotropic therapy in cardiogenic shock.

Monitoring: Arterial blood pressure, heart rate and continuous ECG.

Side effects: Tachycardia, arrhythmias, hypertension.

Administration: When used as an infusion, adrenaline should be infused via a central line because of the risk of vasoconstriction and extravasation injury

Aminophylline

Pharmacology: Aminophylline is a combination of theophylline and ethylenediamine. This combination has the advantage of increased solubility compared to theophylline. Theophylline is an inhibitor of cyclic adenosine monophosphate (cAMP) phosphodiesterase and is an adenosine receptor antagonist. The most clinically useful pharmacological effect is its potent bronchodilator activity.

Indications: Reversible airways disease, severe acute asthma.

Monitoring: Monitoring of plasma concentrations is necessary as theophylline's pharmacokinetics show large interpatient variation, its metabolism can be altered by other drugs and chemicals, and it has a very narrow therapeutic index.

Side effects: Hypokalaemia (particularly in combination with β_2-receptor agonists), tachycardia, palpitations, gastrointestinal disturbances, arrhythmias and, in overdose, convulsions.

Amiodarone

Pharmacology: Amiodarone is a class III antiarrhythmic drug that is useful in the treatment of supraventricular tachycardia and ventricular arrhythmias. Its main mechanism of action is prolongation of the refractory period. It has the advantage of causing little or no myocardial depression. It acts rapidly when given by intravenous infusion and has a very long elimination half-life, particularly after chronic treatment.

Indications: Treatment of arrhythmias, particularly when other drugs are contraindicated or ineffective.

Monitoring: Liver and thyroid function tests should be performed on prolonged oral therapy and during intravenous therapy. Electrocardiograph and blood pressure monitoring are mandatory.

Side effects: Intravenous amiodarone can produce a drop in blood pressure, particularly if infused too rapidly. Hepatotoxicity, thyroid disturbances, peripheral neuropathy, pulmonary toxicity, corneal micro-deposits and phototoxicity may all occur during chronic therapy.

Administration: Infuse centrally if possible, as peripheral infusions are likely to cause thrombophlebitis. When diluted, amiodarone should not be diluted to below $600\,\mu g/ml$ as it precipitates. Dilute in 5% glucose not 0.8% sodium chloride.

Argipressin (vasopressin)

Pharmacology: Vasopressin is a hormone that is produced in the neuronal cells of the hypothalamic nuclei and stored in the posterior lobe of the pituitary gland. It can also be pharmaceutically prepared as argipressin.

Indications: It is used as a potent vasopressor in septic shock as it causes arterial smooth muscle contraction. It is also used for variceal haemorrhage because of its vasoconstrictive effects. It has antidiuretic properties. Vasopressin vasodilates the pulmonary circulation, decreasing pulmonary vascular resistance under both normal and hypoxic conditions as a consequence of V_1-receptor-mediated release of nitric oxide from endothelial cells. Pulmonary artery vasodilation occurs with low concentrations of vasopressin.

Monitoring: Arterial blood pressure, heart rate and continuous ECG. Liver function tests (see below).

Side effects:
- Bilirubin levels may increase during vasopressin infusion (though no clear mechanisms are known), so liver function tests should be closely monitored during infusion
- Conflicting data exist regarding vasopressin's effect on splanchnic circulation, gut hypoperfusion and myocardial ischaemia
- **Adult** data suggests that complications related to 'low'-dose vasopressin appear to be infrequent and minor and can be largely avoided by not administering bolus doses or infusion rates above 0.04 U/min (Mutlu & Factor 2004). (Where high-dose vasopressin was used in one study 4/6 patients had cardiac arrest (Holmes et al 2001).) No data exist, however, for the paediatric population
- May lower body temperature.

Administration: Infuse via a central line as vasopressin is a powerful skin vasoconstrictor and extravasation of even a small quantity of this could cause local skin necrosis. Has a short plasma half-life (5–15 min). Rebound hypotension can occur on discontinuation of vasopressin infusion.

Clonidine

Pharmacology: Clonidine is a partial agonist of α_2-adrenergic receptors and at high doses it can also stimulate α_1-receptors. It is traditionally used as a centrally acting antihypertensive agent. More recently it has been used as a sedative and analgesic. Brain and spinal cord α_2-receptor stimulation modulate the response to pain. Clonidine has also been used to prevent and treat drug withdrawal from opiates, benzodiazepines and other narcotic drugs.

Clonidine has beneficial effects in reducing the catecholamine-mediated cardiovascular response to stress, surgery or intubation. Clonidine does not depress the central respiratory drive and does not inhibit gastric motility. Clonidine presents synergistic effects with opioids and is morphine-sparing, so doses of opioids may be reduced.

Indications: Sedation, analgesia or opioid withdrawal. Usually use oral clonidine first, then, if required, use intravenous clonidine and discontinue oral clonidine.

Monitoring: Blood pressure, heart rate, pain and sedation levels.

Side effects: Hypotension and sinus bradycardia.

Oral use for sedation in PICU:
- Test dose of $1\,\mu g/kg$ (if no hypotension, proceed to maintenance therapy 1 h later).
- Maintenance dose of $1–5\,\mu g/kg$ per dose every 8 h
- If clonidine is used for more than 2 weeks, it must be weaned off over a period of days to prevent rebound. If it is used to prevent or treat drug withdrawal, it should be continued for 2–3 days after the opioids have been stopped.

Dose and administration: Start infusion at $0.25\,\mu g/kg/h$. Increase dose if required by $0.1\,\mu g/kg/h$ until adequate sedation is achieved. Most children do not require doses above $1\,\mu g/kg/h$ (max dose is $2\,\mu g/kg/h$). Do not bolus IV clonidine as it may cause acute hypotension. Reduce dose if hypotension occurs and discontinue if marked hypotension or bradycardia occur.

Dinoprostone (prostaglandin E_2)

Pharmacology: Dinoprostone is derived from the unsaturated long-chain fatty acid arachidonic acid by the cyclo–oxygenase enzyme system, and it takes part in the inflammatory cascade. Prostaglandin E_2 has a variety of pharmacological actions, including vascular smooth muscle relaxation, stimulation of uterine contractions, alteration in renal blood flow resulting in diuresis and involvement in inflammatory responses.

Indications: Dinoprostone is most commonly used in paediatrics to maintain the patency of the ductus arteriosus in neonates with congenital heart defects until corrective surgery is possible. Alprostadil (prostaglandin E_1) can also be used for this purpose. Alprostadil is licensed for this indication but is, however, considerably more expensive.

Monitoring: Arterial blood pressure, oxygen saturation; facilities for intubation and ventilation should be available.

Side effects: Intravenous dinoprostone can cause apnoea and respiratory depression. Other side effects include hypotension, flushing, bradycardia, tachycardia and oedema.

Dobutamine

Pharmacology: Dobutamine stimulates β_1-adrenoreceptors to increase cardiac contractility and β_2-adrenoreceptors to cause vasodilation in mesenteric and skeletal vascular beds. It also stimulates α_1-adrenoreceptors to cause vasoconstriction. The vasodilatory and vasoconstricting effects counterbalance each other and the primary haemodynamic response during dobutamine infusion is an increase in cardiac output, with little change in blood pressure. Dobutamine has no effect upon dopamine receptors.

Indications: Inotropic support in cardiac surgery, cardiomyopathy, septic shock and cardiogenic shock.

Monitoring: Arterial blood pressure, heart rate and continuous ECG.

Side effects: Tachycardia, hypotension, systolic hypertension, arrhythmia, extravasation injury.

Dopamine

Pharmacology: The cardiovascular effects of dopamine are mediated by its stimulation of a number of different receptor types: dopamine D_1 and D_2 receptors; β_1-adrenoreceptors; and α_1-adrenoreceptors.

At low doses (0.5–2 µg/kg/min) the predominant action of dopamine is to stimulate vascular dopamine D_1 receptors, causing vasodilation in mesenteric, renal and coronary vascular beds. The resulting increase in renal blood flow and glomerular filtration rate is the basis of the so called 'renal' dopamine effect. At medium doses (2–5 µg/kg/min) the effects produced by stimulation of β_1-adrenoreceptors are added. Thus, positive inotropic and chronotropic effects usually result in increased systolic blood pressure and pulse pressure with no effect or a small increase in diastolic pressure.

At higher doses (>5 µg/kg/min) dopamine activates α_1-adrenoreceptors, causing vasoconstriction. Thus, increases in systemic vascular resistance, systolic and diastolic blood pressure and a reduced renal dopamine effect are seen.

Indications: Inotropic therapy in cardiogenic shock, and to promote renal perfusion

Monitoring: Arterial blood pressure, heart rate and continuous ECG.

Side effects: Peripheral vasoconstriction, hypertension, tachycardia, extravasation injury.

Enoximone

Pharmacology: Enoximone is a selective inhibitor of phosphodiesterase III (PDEIII). This is the enzyme that is responsible for catalysing the breakdown of cAMP. Inhibition of PDEIII results in accumulation of cAMP. PDEIII is found in high concentrations in cardiac and vascular smooth muscle. Administration of enoximone results in high cAMP levels in cardiac and vascular smooth muscle. This causes positive inotropy and vasodilation. Enoximone is therefore an inodilator.

Indications: Congestive cardiac failure where cardiac output is reduced and filling pressures are increased.

Monitoring: Arterial blood pressure, heart rate and continuous ECG.

Side effects: Arrhythmias, hypotension.

Administration: Infuse centrally or peripherally. It is unstable in solution, only dilute with an equal volume of water for injection or 0.9% saline; do not dilute with any other diluents or use any other concentrations. Do not mix with any other infusions. Enoximone may be given orally.

Furosemide

Pharmacology: Furosemide is a loop diuretic that inhibits electrolyte reabsorption from the ascending limb of the loop of Henle in the renal tubules. It can be useful in renal failure when other groups of diuretics are ineffective but can cause electrolyte disturbances, particularly hypokalaemia. It is one of the most potent diuretics.

Indications: Oedema, oliguria due to renal failure.

Monitoring: Fluid balance, blood urea and electrolytes and blood pressure.

Side effects: Hyponatraemia, hypokalaemia, hypomagnesaemia, hypo-calcaemia, hypotension, hypovolaemia, metabolic acidosis, tinnitus and deafness (particularly in renal failure, large parenteral doses and rapid administration).

Glyceryl trinitrate

Pharmacology: Glyceryl trinitrate produces smooth muscle relaxation and as a result it is a powerful vasodilator of both arterial and venous vas-culature. Its effects are mediated by nitric oxide released when glyceryl trinitrate is metabolised. It is a powerful antihypertensive agent and reduces afterload in cardiac failure. Tolerance to the effects of glyceryl trinitrate often develops after continuous prolonged use.

Indications: Left ventricular failure.

Monitoring: Blood pressure, heart rate, methaemoglobin concentrations.

Side effects: Headache, hypotension, tachycardia, methaemoglobinaemia.

Administration: Nitrates are absorbed on to PVC – select non-PVC syringe and giving set.

Lorazepam

Pharmacology: Lorazepam is a benzodiazepine that has a fast speed of onset and anticonvulsant effects that last up to 24 hours. Other effects include sedation, anxiolysis and amnesia. It does not convert to active metabolites, unlike midazolam. Effects may be reversed by the benzodiazepine antagonist flumazenil, although this is rarely necessary.

Indications: Premedication, sedation with amnesia, status epilepticus.

Monitoring: Blood pressure and oxygen saturation.

Side effects: Hypotension and apnoea – therefore resuscitation facilities should be available.

Administration: IV bolus may be given centrally or peripherally. May be given neat by slow injection.

Midazolam

Pharmacology: Midazolam is a short-acting benzodiazepine that binds to benzodiazepine receptors in the CNS to produce a variety of effects, including sedation, anxiolysis, anticonvulsant effects and amnesia. Effects may be reversed by the benzodiazepine antagonist flumazenil, although this is rarely necessary.

Indications: Sedation, premedication, treatment of epilepsy.

Monitoring: Arterial blood pressure, oxygen saturation.

Side effects: Respiratory depression and severe hypotension after intravenous administration, acute withdrawal syndrome after prolonged use (1–2 weeks). Patients can develop tolerance in 48–72 h.

Milrinone

Pharmacology: Milrinone is a selective inhibitor of phosphodiesterase III, an enzyme responsible for catalysing the breakdown of cAMP. Phosphodiesterase is found in high concentrations in cardiac and vascular smooth muscle. Inhibition of phosphodiesterase results in accumulation of cAMP, which causes positive inotropy and vasodilation. Milrinone is excreted primarily via the kidneys (dose should be reduced in renal failure to avoid accumulation).

Indications: Congestive cardiac failure where cardiac output is reduced and filling pressures are increased. Milrinone acts as an inotrope and afterload reducer.

Monitoring: Arterial blood pressure, heart rate and continuous ECG.

Side effects: Arrhythmias, hypotension.

Dose and administration: Loading dose 50 μg/kg over 10–20 min then infusion rate range 0.3–0.75 μg/kg/min (0.5 μg/kg/min is adequate to maintain therapeutic levels (Bailey et al 1999)). Do not infuse milrinone with furosemide as precipitation occurs. Unlike enoximone, milrinone cannot be given orally.

Morphine

Pharmacology: Morphine is an agonist of a number of morphine receptor subtypes. The most important therapeutic and adverse effects are thought to be mediated via μ and κ opioid receptors. Morphine produces a wide range of pharmacological effects, including analgesia, sedation, respiratory depression, euphoria, inhibition of gut motility, miosis, nausea and vomiting.

Indications: Analgesia, sedation.

Monitoring: Sedation, respiratory rate, oxygen saturation.

Side effects: Nausea and vomiting, constipation, respiratory depression (especially neonates), hypotension, miosis, hallucinations, acute withdrawal syndrome after prolonged use.

Noradrenaline (norepinephrine)

Pharmacology: Noradrenaline is a potent agonist of α-adrenergic receptors. It produces vasoconstriction with an increase in systemic vascular resistance and an elevation of both systolic and diastolic blood pressure. Cardiac output is usually unchanged or reduced. Blood flow to most vascular beds is reduced, including the kidney and the liver.

Indications: Acute hypotension.

Monitoring: Arterial blood pressure, heart rate and continuous ECG.

Side effects: Hypertension, arrhythmias, peripheral ischaemia.

Propofol

Pharmacology: Propofol is a short-acting general anaesthetic agent with a rapid onset of action of approximately 30 s. Propofol reduces cerebral blood flow, intracranial pressure and cerebral metabolism.

Propofol has a rapid distribution with a half-life of 2–4 min and rapid elimination. It is cleared by metabolic processes mainly in the liver and excreted in the urine.

Indications: Sedation, anaesthesia.

Monitoring: Continuous ECG, oxygen saturations and blood pressure. Propofol is formulated in intralipid, so monitor blood lipid levels of all patients.

Side effects: Bradycardia, hypotension, desaturation. Propofol syndrome is a rare and often fatal condition described in children treated with propofol for more than 2–3 d at high doses (>4 mg/kg/h). Symptoms include cardiac failure, rhabdomyolysis, severe lactic acidosis, renal failure and coma.

Administration: IV infusion is not recommended by the Committee on Safety of Medicines; however, if strictly necessary, IV infusion for sedation can be cautiously administered at 2–3 mg/kg/h or adjust dose according to response. Infusion should not continue for more than 2 d and should not exceed 5 mg/kg/h.

 Propofol should be avoided in any patient who is allergic to eggs and soybean oil as there is a risk of anaphylaxis.

Prostaglandin E$_2$

See dinoprostone.

Salbutamol

Pharmacology: Salbutamol is a selective β_2-adrenergic receptor agonist. It is useful principally as a bronchodilator, although other effects such as reducing serum potassium are clinically beneficial.

Indications: Acute asthma, renal hyperkalaemia.

Monitoring: ECG, serum potassium, heart rate, oxygen saturation.

Side effects: Peripheral vasodilation, tachycardia, hypokalaemia.

Sodium nitroprusside (Nipride)

Pharmacology: Sodium nitroprusside produces smooth muscle relaxation and as a result it is a powerful vasodilator of both arterial and venous vasculature. It is effective as an antihypertensive and to reduce preload in cardiac failure. Tolerance is less likely to develop after prolonged use of nitroprusside than with other nitrates. Breakdown of nitroprusside results in the production of thiocyanate, which may accumulate after prolonged infusion (after 3 d or earlier in renal failure).

Indications: Hypertensive crisis, left ventricular failure.

Monitoring: Blood pressure, heart rate, methaemoglobin concentrations, serum thiocyanate levels (after 72 h of infusion).

Side effects: Hypotension, headache, tachycardia, symptoms of rapid blood pressure reduction.

Administration: Maximum concentration 1 mg/ml. Protect infusion from light and use an amber giving set.

Vecuronium

Pharmacology: Vecuronium bromide is a non-depolarising neuromuscular blocking agent with a high degree of selectivity for the nicotinic acetylcholine receptors. Its effects may be reversed by the use of an anticholinesterase drug such as neostigmine. Following an intravenous bolus dose, it has an onset of action of about 2 min and lasts for 15–20 min in children and 30–40 min in infants. It rarely causes histamine release and has good cardiovascular stability. Caution in liver and renal impairment.

Indications: Neuromuscular blockade.

Monitoring: Peripheral nerve stimulator; ventilation is mandatory.

Side effects: Recovery time is increased after prolonged use; very rare hypersensitivity reactions.

THERAPEUTIC DRUG MONITORING

Measurement of plasma levels is necessary for a range of drugs with a narrow therapeutic index. These drugs have a minimum therapeutic concentration that is close to their minimum toxic concentration. The target ranges of concentrations for these drugs are displayed in Table 9.5. The receptor selectivity and pharmacological effects produced by commonly used agents are shown in Table 9.4. It may be necessary at times to run intravenous infusions concurrently and, while this should only be practised where absolutely essential, Table 9.6 shows intravenous compatibilities known.

Table 9.5 Therapeutic drug monitoring

Drug	Recommended sample time	Target range	Time to steady state (approx.)	Sample bottle	Notes
Aminophylline	At least 8 h after starting IV dose	10–20 mg/l	24–48 h	Plain (clotted)	Assay is for theophylline
Carbamazepine	Immediately prior to next dose	4–14 mg/l	2–4 weeks after starting then 3–4 d after each dose change	Plain (clotted)	
Digoxin	6 h post-dose	0.8–2.2 μg/l	5–10 d	Plain (clotted)	
Gentamicin 'once daily'	18 h post-dose	<1 mg/l trough	24 h	Plain (clotted)	Resample after 6–12 h if >1 mg/l
Phenobarbital	Before dose	9–25 mg/l in epilepsy	10–14 d	Plain (clotted)	
Phenytoin	IV: 1 h after end of infusion Orally – before dose	10–20 mg/l infants 6–15 mg/l neonates	1–2 weeks (variable)	Plain (clotted)	Seek advice if albumin binding is altered
Vancomycin	Trough: before dose Peak – 1 h after completing infusion	Trough: 5–10 mg/l Peak: 15–30 mg/l	24–36 h	Plain (clotted)	

Source: information collated from Guy's, St Thomas', King's College and University Lewisham Hospitals 2005.

Table 9.6 Intravenous compatibilities.

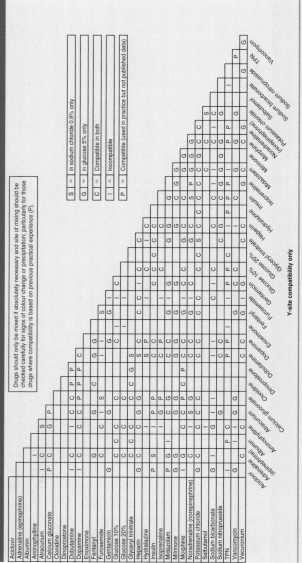

> Drugs should only be mixed if absolutely necessary and site of mixing should be checked carefully for signs of colour change or precipitation; particularly for those drugs where compatibility is based on previous practical experience (P).

Legend:
- S = in sodium chloride 0.9% only
- G = in glucose 5% only
- C = Compatible in both
- I = Incompatible
- P = Compatible (used in practice but not published data)

Y-site compatibility only

Row / column drugs (in order):
Aciclovir; Adrenaline (epinephrine); Albumin; Aminophylline; Atracurium; Calcium gluconate; Clonidine; Dinoprostone; Dobutamine; Dopamine; Enoximone; Fentanyl; Furosemide; Gentamicin; Glucose 10%; Glucose 20%; Glyceryl trinitrate; Heparin; Hydralazine; Insulin; Isoprenaline; Midazolam; Milrinone; Morphine; Noradrenaline (norepinephrine); Potassium chloride; Salbutamol; Sodium bicarbonate; Sodium nitroprusside; TPN; Vancomycin; Vecuronium

Source: with permission from Guy's, St Thomas', King's College and University Lewisham Hospitals (2005).

REFERENCES

Advanced Life Support Group 2006 Advanced Paediatric Life Support: the practical approach, 4th edn. BMJ Publishing Group, London

American Heart Association 1997 Pediatric advanced life support. American Heart Association, Dallas, TX, p 6–9

Bailey JM, Miller BE, Lu W et al 1999 The pharmacokinetics of milrinone in pediatric patients after cardiac surgery. Anesthesiology 90: 1012–1018

Fisher DM 1999 Neuromuscular blocking agents in paediatric anaesthesia. Br J Anaesth 83: 58–64

German DC, Kredich NM, Bjornsson TD 1989 Oral dipyridamole increases plasma adenosine levels in human beings. Clin Pharmacol Ther 45: 80–84

Guy's, St Thomas', King's College and University Lewisham Hospitals 2005 Paediatric formulary, 7th edn. Guy's, St Thomas', King's College and University Lewisham Hospitals, London

Holmes CL, Walley KR, Chittock DR et al 2001 The effects of vasopressin on hemodynamics and renal function in severe septic shock; a case series. Intens Care Med 27: 1416–1421

Mutlu GM, Factor P 2004 Role of vasopressin in the management of septic shock. Intens Care Med 30: 1276–1291

Singer M, Webb A 1997 Oxford handbook of critical care. Oxford University Press, Oxford, p 232

Young LY, Koda-Kimble MA (eds) 1995 Applied therapeutics, 6th edn. Applied Therapeutics, Vancouver, BC

FURTHER READING

Ambrose C, Sale S, Howells R et al 2000 Intravenous clonidine infusion in critically ill children: dose-dependent sedative effects and cardiovascular stability. Br J Anaesth 84: 794–796

Arenas-Lopez S, Riphagen S, Tibby SM 2004 Use of oral clonidine for sedation in ventilated paediatric intensive care patients. Intensive Care Medicine 30: 1625–1629

Royal College of Paediatrics and Child Health 2003 Medicines for children, 2nd edn. Royal College of Paediatrics and Child Health, London

HANDY HINTS FOR VARIOUS CONDITIONS

10

While it is acknowledged that all management will be according to local policies, these guidelines may be helpful.

AIRWAY OBSTRUCTION STRIDOR

Consider the age of the child presenting with stridor (Table 10.1).

Also consider speed of onset as some diagnoses may be more likely (Table 10.2):

- If minutes – foreign body aspiration, anaphylaxis
- If hours – epiglottitis
- If days – croup, mediastinal mass
- If weeks – subglottic stenosis, laryngomalacia, vascular ring.

Table 10.1 Common causes of stridor

Age	Most common causes of stridor
Neonate	Laryngomalacia, vascular ring, subglottic stenosis, laryngeal web
Toddler	Croup, foreign body aspiration, anaphylaxis, epiglottitis
Older child	Mediastinal mass, recurrent croup, acquired subglottic stenosis, anaphylaxis

Table 10.2 Differentiating between epiglottitis and croup

	Epiglottitis	Croup (laryngotracheobronchitis)
Age	2–7 years	1–3 years
History	Hours	1–2 days
Appearance	Toxic, unwell, sits up, mouth open	Anxious, lethargic
Fever	+++ (>38.5°C)	+
Voice	Hoarse, weak	Hoarse
Cough	+	++ (usually barking)
Drooling	+++	Unusual
Respirations	Laboured, stridor	Increased, stridor
Hypoxia	Common	Uncommon

CROUP (LARYNGOTRACHEOBRONCHITIS)

If intubation is required to maintain a secure airway:

- Wean ventilation and allow child to self-ventilate via a Swedish nose filter on the end of the endotracheal (ET) tube
- Secureness of tube is vital – tapes may need to be changed daily because of secretions and movement of child
- Use of arm splints effective in preventing self-extubation
- Regular suction – if child is active, likely to cough up secretions frequently
- Child is likely to be on a course of steroids from admission to PICU – wait to hear leak around tube prior to extubation, can take 3–5 days
- Importance of play, involvement of family in care and daily routine to minimise distress and boredom while ET tube is in situ.

EPIGLOTTITIS

Epiglottitis is most often caused by *Haemophilus influenzae* so is quite rare now the Hib vaccine has been introduced. If a diagnosis of epiglottitis is made, the child will require immediate assessment by a senior anaesthetist or someone who can perform advanced airway procedures, probable intubation under gas induction of anaesthesia, and intravenous antibiotics.

FOREIGN BODY ASPIRATION

History: Usually sudden-onset cough and stridor; however, the act of inhalation may not have been witnessed.

Examination: Often child appears well and active, has stridor and may have wheeze, has differential air entry, may have signs of pneumonia if delayed presentation. Chest X-ray may show differential-hyperinflation.

BACTERIAL TRACHEITIS

Often presents with symptoms similar to croup, but this is a much more serious illness and the child will develop pyrexia and become more unwell. When this child is intubated, pus may be observed in the airway. Intravenous antibiotics will be required.

PRECAUTIONS AND ACTION IN UPPER AIRWAY OBSTRUCTION

- Avoid unnecessary stress for the child, let her/him sit with parents/carers
- Avoid blood gases and X-ray if this will cause distress

- Give oxygen to maintain oxygen saturations prior to intubation
- Give adrenaline (epinephrine) nebulisers (1:1000)
- Give budesonide nebulisers (1 mg total dose)
- Intravenous antibiotics if required
- Advanced airway intervention is a clinical decision

If child requires intubation:

- Call ENT team prior to start
- Use most experienced anaesthetist/operator
- Gas induction in theatre
- Have a wide range of ET tubes ready, especially smaller sizes
- Have a bougie to hand
- Anticipate potential need for a surgical airway.

 Avoid muscle relaxants until the airway is secure.

MANAGEMENT OF SEVERE ASTHMA

Asthmatics have:

- Airway inflammation with wall thickening and increased vascular permeability
- Mucus hypersecretion
- Bronchial smooth muscle contraction (wheeze).

This leads to air trapping and atelectasis. Increased intrathoracic pressure induced by air trapping can reduce cardiac output (tamponade effect).

It is essential to assess the severity of symptoms correctly (Table 10.3) before a child can be effectively treated.

The principles of therapy include:

- Eliminate symptoms and improved lung function
- Correct hypoxia
- Reverse inflammation with steroids
- Relieve smooth muscle constriction with bronchodilators
- If required, supportive ventilation.

Management of asthma

- Nebulised salbutamol 2.5 mg with oxygen as driving gas (repeat if necessary)
- Nebulised ipratropium bromide 0.25 mg

Table 10.3   Assessing severity of asthma

Age	Moderate asthma	Severe asthma	Life-threatening asthma
2–5 years	SpO$_2$ > 92% No clinical features of severe asthma	SpO$_2$ < 92% Too breathless to talk or eat HR > 130 RR > 50 Use of accessory neck muscles	SpO$_2$ < 92% Silent chest Poor resp. effort Agitation Altered LOC Cyanosis
>5 years	SpO$_2$ > 92% Peak flow > 50% best or predicted No clinical features of severe asthma	SpO$_2$ < 92% Peak flow < 50% best or predicted HR > 120 RR > 30 Use of accessory neck muscles	SpO$_2$ < 92% Peak flow < 33% best or predicted Silent chest Poor resp. effort Altered LOC Cyanosis

HR, heart rate; LOC, level of consciousness; RR, respiratory rate.
Source: from British Thoracic Society 2003.

- IV hydrocortisone 4 mg/kg
- High-flow oxygen mask with reservoir if S$_p$O$_2$ < 92%.

If worsening respiratory distress or no improvement in severe or life-threatening categories, progress to:

- IV salbutamol infusion 1–5 µg/kg/min (consider bolus IV salbutamol 15 µg/kg of 200 µg/ml solution over 10 min; British Thoracic Society 2004)
- Consider IV magnesium sulphate 40 mg/kg (max. 2 g) of 50% solution over 20 min. One dose only (Ciarallo et al 2000).

Magnesium sulphate is contraindicated in renal failure. Magnesium sulphate may induce moderate hypotension and muscle weakness.

- Consider IV aminophylline 1 mg/kg/h after bolus of 5 mg/kg over 20 min (unless receiving oral theophyllines)
- IV antibiotics if focal areas on chest X-ray.

Monitor serum potassium if salbutamol is used and give potassium supplements if serum potassium is low.

Criteria for intubation (Phipps & Garrard 2003, Biaret 1999)

- Exhaustion, respiratory muscle fatigue
- Decreased chest movement with breathing
- Quiet chest, absent audible wheeze
- Pulsus paradoxus (systolic pressure >20 mmHg)
- Lethargy, agitation, confusion, coma
- Severe mucous plugging and lobar collapse
- Profound hypoxaemia

 Avoid paralysing agents such as atracurium for intubation as they cause histamine release. (Could use vecuronium or rocuronium, for example, with ketamine for intubation.)

Strategies for ventilation

- Suggested initial settings – tidal volume 6–8 ml/kg or peak inspiratory pressure (PIP) to generate chest movement, low rate, e.g. 12 breaths/min, inspiratory time 1.0, I:E ratio 1:3 or 1:4, positive end–expiratory pressure (PEEP) 5, F_iO_2 0.6
- Humidification essential, plus regular ET suction
- Permissive hypercapnia, permissive hypoxia to avoid barotrauma (sats >88%, pH >7.2)
- May require high levels of sedation while ventilated
- Switch to pressure support ventilation mode as soon as possible.

Peak pause pressures

Airflow obstruction in asthma can be quantified by a peak inspiratory pause manoeuvre by closing the inspiratory valve at the end of inspiration (i.e. holding the pause knob on the Servo ventilator). This results in a full breath being delivered into the lungs. In 'normal' lungs, there will be no drop in the PIP after an inspiratory pause because there is no change in flow (i.e. no obstruction in the airways). In asthma, pressure will be dissipated by overcoming the resistance in the major airways due to obstruction to airflow by bronchospasm or mucus plugs. As a result, a fall in pressure will occur on inflation of the lungs, reaching a plateau only when airflow resistance is overcome. This fall in pressure (from peak to plateau pressures) is proportional to airway resistance.

AutoPEEP can be measured by an expiratory hold manoeuvre (closing the expiratory valve on expiration). This will be positive if airflow is still occurring at the end of expiration (i.e. the alveoli are still emptying). The higher the expiratory pause pressure (autoPEEP), the higher the flow limitation during expiration. It has been suggested that low-level externally applied PEEP (<7.5 cmH₂O) may overcome the obstruction to flow without increasing alveolar pressure.

Crisis management

- Hand–ventilate 100% oxygen, no PEEP for 1 min giving only very low rate
- Ketamine infusion (bronchial smooth muscle dilator)
- Isoflurane/heliox administration via ventilator
- Extracorporeal membrane oxygenation (ECMO).

 Anticipate arrhythmias, barotraumas and hypotension due to over-distension – treat with volume.

DIABETIC KETOACIDOSIS

Diabetic ketoacidosis (DKA) is a state of hypertonic dehydration and metabolic decompensation that results from inadequate levels of insulin in the body.

- Problems include: hyperglycaemia, ketoacidaemia, acid–base disturbance, electrolyte disturbances
- Leading causes of death in children with DKA:
  - Cerebral oedema

Box 10.1 Risk factors for cerebral oedema

- Younger age
- P_{CO_2} < 2 kPa at presentation (Glaser et al 2001)
- pH < 7.1 at presentation (Mahoney et al 1999, Roberts et al 2001)
- >40 ml/kg IV fluid in first 4 h (Roberts et al 2001)
- Rapid falls in corrected sodium (Mahoney et al 1999)
- NaHCO$_3$ therapy (Glaser et al 2001)
- Raised serum urea (Glaser et al 2001)
- Hyperventilation post intubation.

Box 10.2 Principles of therapy

- Treatment of shock (do not treat capillary refill)
- Correction of ketoacidosis (insulin ± dextrose)
- **Slow** rehydration over 48 h
- Avoidance of cerebral oedema
- Replacement of K$^+$ and PO$_4$
- **Continuous careful monitoring.**

- Hypokalaemia
- Inhalation of vomit

- Airway – Breathing – Circulation.

Diabetic ketoacidosis with cerebral oedema: management strategy

This is one guideline that is current and referenced, but the authors recognise that opinions vary so consult local guidelines and protocols.

Monitoring on therapy

- Glasgow Coma Scale and neuro–observations should be monitored every half-hour
- Glucose (BM) hourly
- 2-hourly
  - U+E, PO_4, lab. glucose and osmolality
  - ABG, anion gap and Cl:Na ratio
  - Calculate Corrected Sodium
  - Urine Dipstix (must have glucose and ketones if DKA)
- Catheter and nasogastric tube should be placed for accurate fluid balance (**do not** chase urine output).

Corrected sodium (Na corr.)

Plasma (Na) $+ 0.4$ ([Glucose] $- 5.5$)

Anion gap

$$([Na] + [K]) - ([Cl] + [HCO_3]): \text{normal} <18\,\text{mEq/l}.$$

(Anion gap should resolve within 20 hours; otherwise consider other potential diagnosis, including sepsis).

PROTOCOL

Resuscitation

1. Avoid fluid boluses unless hypotensive (max. 20 ml/kg in first 4 h)
2. Use inotropes (dopamine) if hypotensive despite 20 ml/kg fluid boluses
3. Consider 3% saline (2 ml/kg) if refractory hypotension or cerebral oedema suspected
4. Remember antibiotics if sepsis suspected
5. **Do not** chase capillary refill times
6. Account for excessive fluid resuscitation in rehydration.

Fig 10.1   Two-bag system

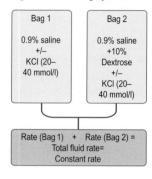

- **Total fluid rate is the sum of the infusion rates of Bags 1 and 2 and must be constant:**
  Rate (Bag 1) + Rate (Bag 2) = Total fluid rate = Constant
- The aim is to steadily reduce then stabilise blood glucose without changing the insulin dose
- Initial fluid will usually be Bag 1 (normal saline *without* added dextrose)
- Start Bag 2 (normal saline *with* 10% dextrose) when:
  - Glucose <15 mmol/l or
  - Glucose falls >5 mmol/l/h or
- As blood glucose changes adjust ratio of Bag 1 to Bag 2 to try and produce a steady fall (<5 mmol/l/h) then keep BM 8–12 mmol/l
- **Do not stop the insulin** if glucose falls. It may be *reduced* (to 0.05 IU/kg/h when anion gap <18)

Try to manage patient condition without placing central lines if possible, as in DKA there is increased incidence of thrombosis.

Ketoacidosis

1. Ketosis only resolves with insulin therapy. Start insulin at 0.1 U/kg/h 2.5 × wt (kg) units insulin (Actrapid) in 50 ml 0.9% saline gives 1 ml/h as 0.05 U/kg/h
2. Follow resolution of ketosis by measuring anion gap (calculate)
   a. Base excess and pH may be unreliable, as hyperchloraemic acidosis develops on saline (indicated by persisting base deficit with Cl:Na ratio >0.78 and anion gap <18)
   b. Urine ketones usually persist for 24–48 hours and **do not** reflect serum ketonaemia
   c. **Do not** reduce insulin until anion gap <18 mmol/l (ketosis resolved)
3. When serum glucose <15 mmol/l, introduce glucose via the two-bag system (Poirier et al 2004; Fig. 10.1)
4. Insulin reduces serum K^+ – add to all fluid bags as KCl unless $[K^+]$ >5.5 mmol/l.
5. Supplement PO_4^- (<0.6 mmol/l) as separate KPO_4 IV infusion (over 6 h).

Table 10.4 Total intravenous fluid requirements in diabetic ketoacidosis

Weight (kg)	Total fluid rate
0–9.9	4 ml/kg/h
10–39.9	3 ml/kg/h
>40	2 ml/kg/h

This includes maintenance and 10% rehydration.

Fig 10.2 Any fall in corrected sodium associated with headache, agitation or decreased Glasgow Coma Scale should be treated with 3% saline

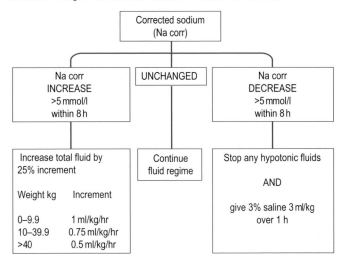

Maintenance and rehydration (total fluid rate)

1. **Always rehydrate over 48 h** (we assume ICU patients are 10% dehydrated)
2. **Always give isotonic fluid** (0.9% saline ±10% dextrose) regardless of plasma [Na]. However if BM > 15 mmol/l, just give 0.9% saline
3. Prescribe hourly total fluid rate according to Table 10.4 over 48 h.
4. If more than 40 ml/kg resus fluid given decrease total fluid rate by 25%
5. **Do not** chase urine output
6. Commence enteral feeds when ketones have disappeared
7. **Adjust fluid rate only according to Na corr** (Fig. 10.2).

Depressed consciousness – always assume cerebral oedema

1. Always discuss the patient with the consultant on call
2. Osmotherapy is the first line
   Give 3 ml/kg 3% saline (whatever the serum sodium), or 0.5 g/kg mannitol (2.5 ml/kg of 20% mannitol) if this not available
3. If the patient does not respond to this or it is not protecting the airway:
   a. Intubate and ventilate (aim for normal P_{CO_2} 4–4.5 kPa)
   b. Computed tomography scan
   c. Sedate, head-up 30°, and neuroprotect

(Dan Taylor, Guy's Hospital PICU).

BURNS

Of the 5000–6000 burned or scalded children requiring hospital admission each year (Advanced Life Support Group 2005) it is believed that fewer than 100 will need admission to PICU (Stack & Dobbs 2004). Most fatal burns occur in house fires and the usual cause of death is smoke inhalation (Advanced Life Support Group 2005).

The National Burn Care Review (National Burn Care Review Committee 2001) recommends that children with burns should be treated in a burns centre.

Criteria for transfer to a burns unit:
- 10% partial and/or full thickness burns
- 5% full thickness burns
- Burns to special areas (face/hands/feet/perineum)
- Any circumferential burn
- Significant inhalational burn (excluding pure carbon monoxide poisoning)
- Chemical, radiation or high voltage electrical burn (Advanced Life Support Group 2005).

Box 10.3 Indications of inhalational injury

- History of exposure to smoke in a confined space
- Deposits around mouth and nose
- Carbonaceous sputum.
  Immediately consider need for tracheal intubation (Advanced Life Support Group 2005)

Four main categories:

- Thermal
- Chemical
- Electrical
- Radiation.

Airway – Breathing – Circulation – Disability – Exposure

- **Airway** may be compromised due to inhalational injury or severe burns to the face. Direct inhalational injury causes damage to mucosa and underlying tissues. The resultant oedema carries the risk of airway obstruction. If there is any suspicion of cervical spine injury/history is unobtainable, take appropriate precautions until such history is excluded (Advanced Life Support Group 2005)
- **Breathing** may be compromised by circumferential burns to the chest, which may mechanically restrict breathing. Indirect inhalational injury – smoke inhalation may cause inflammation and ulceration in the upper airway, trachea and large bronchi. Risk of pneumonia and ARDS developing 24–48 h post injury. High-frequency oscillation may be considered if difficult to ventilate, to reduce the risk of barotrauma. Carbon monoxide from smoke combines with haemoglobin to form carboxy-haemoglobin (COHb), incapable of transporting O_2 to the tissues. Assess COHb level by co-oximeter reading. S_aO_2 may be ineffective – normal readings may occur despite reduced content of O_2 in the blood. O_2 reduces the half life of CO from 5–6 h to 1.5 h in 100% O_2.

 All children who have suffered a burn injury should be given high flow/100% O_2.

- **Circulation** In the first few hours following injury, signs of hypovolaemic shock are rarely attributable to burns – any such signs should therefore raise the suspicion of bleeding from elsewhere and the source should be actively sought (Advanced Life Support Group 2005). Fluid resuscitation should be administered following assessment of the burn. Inotropes may be indicated in children with burns covering more than 30–40% total body surface area (TBSA).

Assessment of the burn

Two main factors:

- Percentage of the TBSA
- Depth.

Fig 10.3   Lund & Browder chart to calculate percentage of total body surface area (courtesy of Smith & Nephew Pharmaceuticals Ltd)

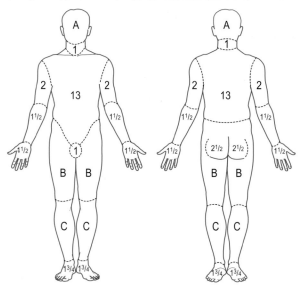

Also consider special areas:

- Face and mouth
- Hands and feet,
- Perineal area.

Total body surface area

- Estimate using burn chart – Lund & Browder commonly used (Fig. 10.3)
- Important to use a paediatric chart as surface area of head and limbs change with age (Table 10.5)
- Child's palm and adducted fingers form approximately 1% of their TBSA
- Note that Rule of Nines does not apply to a child under the age of 14 years.

Table 10.5 Surface area of legs and head at different ages

Area (see Fig. 10.3)	Birth	1 year	5 years	10 years	15 years
		Surface area (%) at:			
A	9.5	8.5	6.5	5.5	4.5
B	2.75	3.25	4.0	4.5	4.5
C	2.5	2.5	2.75	3.0	3.25

Source: with permission from Advanced Life Support Group 2005.

Box 10.4   Parkland formula

4 ml × weight (kg) × %TBSA burned to be given in the first 24 h:

- 50% given in the first 8 h from time of injury
- 50% given over remaining 16 h.

Depth

- **Superficial** Injury to epidermis: skin appears red with no blister formation
- **Partial thickness** Some change to dermis, skin is pink or mottled, blisters usually seen
- **Full thickness** Damage to both epidermis and dermis and may cause damage to deeper structures. Skin appears white, charred, is painless and leathery to touch.

Escharotomies may need to be undertaken in the event of circumferential burns to prevent compartment syndrome.

Fluid management

Fluid is required for:

- Resuscitation
- Normal maintenance
- Burned area when the burn comprises more than 10% of the TBSA. This additional fluid can be estimated using the Parkland formula (Box 10.4).

Fluid given is usually crystalloid (Hartmanns/0.9% saline). Evaluation is largely based on urine output – catheterise as soon as possible and aim for at least 1 ml/kg/h – in addition to vital signs, acid–base balance and lactate.

Wound management

- Major risk of infection
- Wounds may be cleaned using 0.9% saline and initially covered with sterile towels/cling film
- Adhere to local policies/advice from burns centre re dressings used
- Avoid heat loss
- Culture regularly and treat identified infections with appropriate antibiotics
- Surgical intervention – may include skin grafting.

Nutrition management

Enteral feeds should be introduced as soon as possible – monitor weight, calorie and protein intake. Various formulae used to calculate daily requirements.

Pain management

- Ensure effective analgesia provided by continuous opiate infusion
- Organise psychological support for child and carers.

Electrocution

- Deep burn through tissues
- Entry and exit wounds
- Cardiac arrest common
- Ventricular fibrillation precipitated by current through heart
- Primary respiratory arrest or asphyxiation due to chest wall tetany
- Loss of consciousness or seizures
- Acute renal failure due to myoglobin or direct electrical injury
- Haemorrhage and thrombosis.

Management

- Cardiopulmonary resuscitation
- Fluid to maintain good urine output, often requiring more than expected for the surface burn area
- Fasciotomy of damaged area (Stack & Dobbs 2004).

MENINGOCOCCAL MENINGITIS

Fig 10.4(a) Early management of meningococcal sepsis – an evidence-based guideline

Pathology

- 60% children present with features of both meningitis and septicaemia
- 20% children present with meningitis alone
- Approx 20% children present with septicaemia alone (Schildkamp 1996)
- Approx 20% children have no rash on presentation
- Most children present with purpuric/petechial non-balancing rash

Extensive or rapidly spreading rash usually indicates severe disease (Baines & Hart 2003)

Signs of shock

Septic shock can be identified BEFORE hypotension occurs by triad; hypo or hyperthermia, altered mental status, peripheral vasodilation (warm shock) or cool extremities (cold shock) (Carcillo et al 2002)

Signs of early compensated shock include:
tachycardia, cool peripheries, increased capillary refill time tachypnoea/pulse oximetry <95%, hypoxia on ABG, base deficit (worse than – 5 mmol/l), confusion, poor urine output (<1ml/kg/h)

Hypotension is a late sign (Pollard et al 1999)

Principles of therapy

- Protect airway
- Prompt treatment of shock
- Appropriate ventilatory management
- Management of raised ICP
- Frequent reassessment of ABCD
CONTINUOUS CAREFUL
MONITORING

EARLY INTUBATION HAS BEEN
SHOWN TO IMPROVE SURVIVAL

To run simultaneously with ABCD assessment

- Obtain IV access 2x large bore peripheral cannulae or I/O access if unable to gain peripheral access
- Take arterial blood gas, blood sugar, lactate, urea and electrolytes, liver function tests, CRP, full blood count, clotting screen, x-match, blood culture, inform public health.
- **GIVE ANTIBIOTICS ASAP** – ceftriaxone 80 mg/kg intravenously to all ages, as soon as possible, except in confirmed cephalosporin allergy. In this case give ciprofloxacin (or rifampicin if under 6 years).
- Site arterial line and central venous line (if required for inotropes)
- Nasogastric tube
- Catheterise
- Chest X-ray
- Check for and correct – hypoglycaemia (aim to maintain blood sugar levels in normal range (Hotchkiss & Karl 2003, Van den Berghe et al 2003). hypokalaemia (give 0.5 mmol/kg), hypomagnesemia (give 100 mg/kg, max 10ml)
- Blood products. Give fresh frozen plasma (10–20 ml/kg) for coagulaopathy ie prolonged prothrombin time; but beware this may cause hypotension due to vasoactive kinins. Give cryoprecipitate (5ml/kg) if fibrinogen < 1g/l. Packed cells to maintain Hb >10 g/dl. Give platelets if <50 or if bleeding.
- Active temperature control with paracetamol and cooling. Rectal temperature reading may be inaccurate because of splanchnic hypoperfusion
- Guide for systolic BP in children = 80 + (age in years x2). Note trends in vital signs rather than absolute values

ABCD assessment

High-flow face mask O₂. Intubate if:
- cardiac or respiratory arrest or
- after 40–60 ml/kg fluid resuscitation and still signs of shock or
- AVPU – not responding to voice or
- if hypoxic on ABG or
- if signs of ↑ICP (ie ↑BP, relative bradycardia, pupil signs)

Avoid nasal intubation if clotting deranged. Use ketamine 1–2 mg/kg and vecuronium 80–100 μg/kg for intubation,
(Have fluid bolus prepared to give if required)

If self-ventilating, monitor tachypnoea and work of breathing, ensure saturations ? 95%. If signs of shock, give 20 ml/kg crystalloid fluid stat and review (Alderson et al 2003).

Repeat 20 ml/kg x2 crystalloid bolus if no or minimal response. Review. Assess central and peripheral pulses. Inotropes may now be required. Assess pupils for size, reaction to light and position. If fixed and dilated or asymmetrical, give bolus 3 ml/kg 3% saline (Qureshi & Suarez 2000)

Do not perform lumbar puncture (Rennick 1993)

Fig 10.4(b) Early management of meningococcal sepsis – an evidence-based guideline (*continued*)

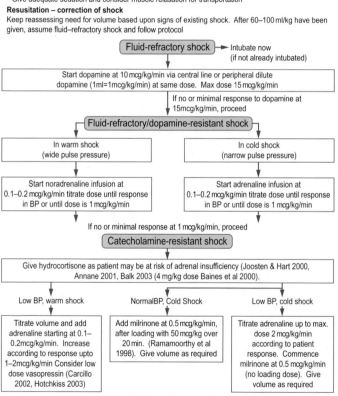

Review airway, breathing, circulation and neurostatus frequently.

Protocol

Acute lung injury/pulmonary oedema ventilation strategy
- Hypoxia → Fio₂ 1.0 initially
- Recruitment manoeuvres
- High PEEP
- Accept Sao₂ ? 92%
- Permissive hypercapnia
- Consider low tidal volumes 6 ml/kg ventilation (Vincent et al 2002)
- Give adequate sedation and consider muscle relaxation for transportation

Resuscitation – correction of shock
Keep reassessing need for volume based upon signs of existing shock. After 60–100 ml/kg have been given, assume fluid–refractory shock and follow protocol

Fluid-refractory shock → Intubate now
(if not already intubated)

Start dopamine at 10 mcg/kg/min via central line or peripheral dilute dopamine (1ml=1mcg/kg/min) at same dose. Max dose 15 mcg/kg/min

If no or minimal response to dopamine at 15mcg/kg/min, proceed

Fluid-refractory/dopamine-resistant shock

In warm shock (wide pulse pressure)	In cold shock (narrow pulse pressure)
Start noradrenaline infusion at 0.1–0.2 mcg/kg/min titrate dose until response in BP or until dose is 1 mcg/kg/min	Start adrenaline infusion at 0.1–0.2 mcg/kg/min titrate dose until response in BP or until dose is 1 mcg/kg/min

If no or minimal response at 1 mcg/kg/min, proceed

Catecholamine-resistant shock

Give hydrocortisone as patient may be at risk of adrenal insufficiency (Joosten & Hart 2000, Annane 2001, Balk 2003 (4 mg/kg dose Baines et al 2000).

Low BP, warm shock	NormalBP, Cold Shock	Low BP, cold shock
Titrate volume and add adrenaline starting at 0.1–0.2mcg/kg/min. Increase according to response upto 1–2mcg/kg/min Consider low dose vasopressin (Carcillo 2002, Hotchkiss 2003)	Add milrinone at 0.5 mcg/kg/min, after loading with 50 mcg/kg over 20 min. (Ramamoorthy et al 1998). Give volume as required	Titrate adrenaline up to max. dose 2 mcg/kg/min according to patient response. Commence milrinone at 0.5 mcg/kg/min (no loading dose). Give volume as required

Titrate adrenaline and noradrenaline up to max. dose of 2 mcg/kg/min according to response. If minimal or no response reassess need for more fluid

Reassess ABCD

Consider calcium infusion for refractory hypotension (Baines 2003)
Consider other unrecognised morbidities, e.g. pericardial effusion, pneumothorax, ongoing blood loss, intra-abdominal catastrophe

REFERENCES

Advanced Life Support Group 2005 Advanced Paediatric Life Support: a practical approach, 4th edn. BMJ, London

Alderson P et al 2003 Colloids versus crystalloids for fluid resuscitation in critically ill patients (Cochrane Review). In: The Cochrane Library, Issue 3, Oxford: Update Software

Annane D 2001 Corticosteroids for septic shock. Crit Care Med 29: S117–S120

Baines PB, Hart CA 2003 Severe meningococcal disease in childhood. Br J Anaesth 90: 72–83

Balk RA 2003 Steroids for septic shock: back from the dead. Chest: 123: 490S–499S

Biaret D 1999 Mechanical ventilation in asthma. Available on line at: http://picuBOOK.net/1999/04-12a

British Thoracic Society 2003 British guidelines for the management of asthma. Thorax 58(Suppl)

British Thoracic Society 2004 British guideline on the management of asthma. British Thoracic Society/Scottish Intercollegiate Guidelines Network, London

Carcillo JA, Fields AI, Task Force Committee Members 2002 Clinical practice parameters for hemodynamic support of pediatric and neonatal patients in septic shock. J Pediatr 78: 449–466

Ciarallo L, Brousseau D, Reinert S 2000 Higher-dose intravenous magnesium therapy for children with moderate to severe asthma. Arch Pediatr Adolesc Med 154: 979–983

Glaser N, Barnett P, McCaslin I et al 2001 Risk factors for cerebral oedema in children with diabetic ketoacidosis. N Engl J Med 344: 264–269

Hotchkiss RS, Karl IE 2003 Medical progress: the pathophysiology and treatment of sepsis. N Engl J Med 348: 138–150

Joosten KFM, de Kleijn ED, Westerterp M et al 2000 Endocrine and metabolic responses in children with meningococcal sepsis: striking differences between survivors and nonsurvivors. J Clin Endocrinol Metab 85: 3746–3753

Mahoney CP, Vlcek BW, DelAguila M 1999 Risk factors for developing brain herniation during diabetic ketoacidosis. Pediatr Neurol 21: 721–727

National Burn Care Review Committee 2001 National burn care review: standards and strategy for burn care. British Association of Plastic Surgeons, London

Phipps P, Garrard CS 2003 The pulmonary physician in critical care. 12: Acute, severe asthma in the intensive care unit. Thorax 58: 81–88

Poirier MP et al 2004 A prospective study of the two bag system in diabetic ketoacidosis management. Clin Pediatr 43: 809–813

Pollard AJ, Britto J, Nadel S et al 1999 Emergency management of meningococcal disease. Arch Dis Childh 80: 290–296

Qureshi S, Suarez J 2000 Use of hypertonic saline solutions in the treatment of cerebral edema and intracranial hypertension. Crit Care Med 28: 3301–3313

Ramamoorthy C, Anderson GD, Williams GD, Lynn AM 1998 Pharmacokinetics and side effects of milrinone in infants and children after open heart surgery. Anesth Analg 86: 283–289

Rennick G, Shann F, de Campo J 1993 Cerebral herniation during bacterial meningitis in children. Br Med J 306: 953–955

Roberts MD, Slover RH, Chase HP 2001 Diabetic ketoacidosis with intracerebral complications. Pediatr Diabetes 2: 109–114

Schildkamp RL, Lodder MC, Bijlmer HA et al 1996 Clinical manifestations and course of meningococcal disease in 562 patients. Scand J Infect Dis 28: 47–51

Stack C, Dobbs P 2004 Essentials of paediatric intensive care. Greenwich Medical, London

Van den Berghe G, Wouters PJ, Bouillon R et al, 2003 Outcome benefit of intensive insulin therapy in the critically ill: Insulin dose versus glycaemic control. Crit Care Med 31: 359–366

11

Lead centre PICUs should have a fully equipped, resourced retrieval service available 24 hours a day, 7 days a week for children who require intensive care within an agreed catchment area whenever a bed is required (Department of Health 1997a, Paediatric Intensive Care Society 2001). The British Paediatric Association (1993) identified the need for a specialised team for the transfer of critically ill children. The dangers of non-specialised paediatric transfers highlighted serious clinical complications in three-quarters of patients transferred, almost one-quarter of which were considered life-threatening (Barry & Ralston 1994). The Paediatric Intensive Care Society standards (2001) describe a doctor and nurse team as suitable personnel to carry out a retrieval. However, a growing number of centres around the world use advanced or extended practice nurses for all or most of their paediatric transports (King & Woodward 2001), with no medical personnel unless for training purposes. There are currently advanced nurse practitioners being trained in the UK to fulfil this role. The government's document *Framework for the Future* (Department of Health 1997a), states: '[T]he most important element, by far, is the skills and experience of the medical and nursing staff who will be caring for the critically ill child'. These advanced nurse practitioners must be aware that the standards of care apply to a task, not a person, so that inexperience is no defence in the eyes of the law (Melville & Print 1996).

The retrieval service must provide 'an intensive care bed on the move' (Paediatric Intensive Care Society 1996), which should include compact, mobile and reliable monitoring and therapy in transit. There is no specific documentation required by law during interhospital transfer but the record must reflect the condition, treatment, care received and response of the patient (Melville & Print 1996).

New European standards for ambulance vehicles and their equipment were recommended by the European Committee for Standardisation (CEN) in 1999. These European standards specify requirements for the design, testing, performance and equipping of road ambulances used in the transportation of the sick child, including the provision of medical devices. Adequate insurance for all members of the retrieval team must be provided by the trust where the team is based.

THE RETRIEVAL NURSE

It is acknowledged that the participation of nursing staff as members of the transfer team is essential: they act as skilled assistants to the team leader/medical staff and are able to assess the nursing needs of the child (Paediatric Intensive Care Society 2001). It is important that only experienced and appropriately trained nurses take on this role as a wide range of skills and expertise are required, in a difficult working environment without the assistance of colleagues. A confident, competent practitioner is required who can cope with the considerable demands of the role, and familiarity with the *Scope of Professional Practice* (UKCC 1992) is essential. It is recommended that only nurses with a higher qualification in paediatric intensive care – the ENB 415 or equivalent – should participate and that, in addition, in-house training should be provided for all those participating in retrievals (Department of Health 1997b, Paediatric Intensive Care Society 2001).

COMMUNICATION

One of the key skills required for a retrieval team to function smoothly and effectively is good communication; this is particularly important among the staff members of the retrieval team enabling efficient teamwork to take place. This team then needs to communicate effectively with its base, the ambulance crew, the child and family and the staff at the referring hospital. Forming friendly, constructive relationships with the staff who have recognised the need to transfer the child to your unit and may have worked hard for many hours resuscitating and trying to stabilise a sick child is very important.

As well as training their own staff, it is envisaged that Lead Centres should develop into a resource providing advice and training covering their whole geographical area; by arranging placements for both doctors and nurses from centres that see relatively few critically ill children, opportunities for them to maintain their skills will be provided (Department of Health 1997a).

BEFORE YOU LEAVE

- All equipment should have been checked; monitors and pumps should be fully charged
- Consider the age, size and provisional diagnosis of the child – do you need to take anything extra or, alternatively, could you leave anything behind? For example, if you are retrieving an infant, do you really need to take a range of large ET tubes just because they are part of the standard kit?
- Regardless of the contents of your kit, many people find it invaluable to have scissors, a few plain labels, pens, a calculator and a roll of clear tape in their pockets
- The doctor will have discussed the child with staff at the referring unit and possibly given them advice on further management while

they await the team's arrival. Check that the location of the child within the referring hospital is documented, together with directions if appropriate, as this can save valuable time.

ON ARRIVAL

- Assess the child together with your colleague/s – the medical and nursing staff at the referring hospital should provide a history and update on current management
- As soon as you can, locate and introduce yourself briefly to parents/relatives and give them your information booklet
- Liaise closely with the nurse caring for the child. The help of this nurse could be invaluable – s/he knows the child and the layout of the unit. The nurse may be keen to assist you and learn from you, having participated in the management and stabilisation of the child prior to your arrival.

While carrying out your initial assessment of the child, ascertain the following:

- If the child is ventilated, what is the size, length, position and mode of securing of the ET tube?
- Is adequate cervical-spine protection in place if required and appropriate?
- Is the child effectively ventilated or are there problems?
- Were there any problems during intubation and is there a leak around the tube?
- Has a recent arterial blood gas analysis been undertaken?
- Where are chest and other X-rays?
- Is the child cardiovascularly stable? Are the child's heart rate and blood pressure within reasonable ranges for his/her age and condition?
- If the child has had cardiac rhythm disturbances or a cardiac arrest, ascertain if a cause was found, and the treatment required to stabilise the child's condition
- Has a 12-lead ECG been performed, if required?
- Assess the child's current perfusion – central and peripheral pulses and what is the capillary refill time?
- Note peripheral and central lines, their location, patency, secureness of dressings and the fluids/drugs running through them
- Check and record the dosages of drug infusions/fluids in progress, paying particular attention if the patient is a child with a suspected congenital cardiac abnormality on a Prostin E_2 infusion – this drug has been known to be confused with prostacyclin, which could have serious implications and, as the dosage is calculated in nanograms, there is increased potential for error
- Note any allergies

- Note blood/specimen results that may be available
- Has a recent blood sugar level been checked?
- What is the child's urine output like? Quantity/colour/urinalysis?
- Has s/he been catheterised?
- What are the core/peripheral temperatures?
- Does the child have any rash/cuts/bruises/superficial or more serious injuries (e.g. consider abdominal injury)?
- Assess and document the child's neurological status, taking into consideration drugs that have been given or are in progress.

Try to gain some space to lay out the equipment you need – ask to borrow some trolleys, as these are invaluable, enabling you to lay out drugs/equipment for any procedure you need to undertake.

When you have completed all procedures required to stabilise and treat the child, prior to preparing to leave the parents will need to be updated and see their child. They may, of course, be present throughout the stabilisation period. Check their travel arrangements – if they are very shocked/distressed, it is inadvisable for them to drive. If a friend/relative is unable to help them, involve staff at the referring hospital in making arrangements. Many teams provide maps for parents together with their information booklet, to make their journey easier. If the parents are driving, make sure they understand that under no circumstances should they attempt to follow the ambulance as it travels with blue lights at speed back to your base. If traffic is likely to be heavy or the doctor feels it is indicated for other reasons, a police escort may be required, which will need to be organised.

BEFORE TRANSFER

Safety

- Infant or child must be appropriately secured on the transfer trolley or in transport incubator or pod prior to departure
- Appropriate continuous monitoring in situ – ECG, pulse oximetry, continuous/intermittent blood pressure, respiratory rate and heart rate
- Appropriate limits set on transport monitor
- All equipment, including monitor and infusion pumps, must be secured prior to departure
- Physiological variables should be recorded as a baseline at the referring hospital and during the transfer, as well as therapeutic interventions
- Adverse incidents must be documented and reported
- Adequate and appropriate sedation with or without paralysis should be used
- Portable suction working and to hand with appropriate-sized suction catheters.

Airway

- Airway safe or secured by intubation
- Position of endotracheal tube assessed clinically/X-ray prior to departure and well secured
- Humidification in ventilator circuit
- Consider need to suction ET tube prior to departure
- Reintubation equipment, e.g. spare ET tube of same size plus one size smaller, Magill's, laryngoscope, mask and airway to hand for transfer
- Nasogastric or orogastric tube in situ.

Breathing

- Select transport ventilator appropriate for age and weight of patient (preferably with high pressure and disconnect alarms)
- Check adequate gas exchange once stabilised on transport ventilator, confirmed by arterial blood gas if appropriate
- End-tidal CO_2 monitoring in situ
- Adequate supply of oxygen in ambulance and reserve supply for emergency use
- A re-breathe bag and self-inflating bag to hand as a back-up during transfer
- A supply of air for ventilator use if required
- A positive end-expiratory pressure (PEEP) valve in use if required.

Circulation

- Continuous haemodynamic monitoring as previously described
- Ensure at least two intravenous cannulas in situ that have been checked as patent by the retrieval team
- Ensure that intravenous and arterial lines are securely fastened and labelled, with easy access to the intravenous lines during transfer
- If a central venous line is inserted for clinical reasons, it should be monitored
- As far as possible, the child should be haemodynamically stable for transfer but, in situations where ongoing haemodynamic deterioration is likely, e.g. meningococcal septicaemia, appropriate anticipatory measures must be undertaken, e.g. draw up sufficient fluids and inotropic infusions
- Ensure arterial and CVP lines are re-zeroed once transducers have been attached to child
- Most recent blood results documented and appropriate treatment administered as required.

Neurology/trauma

- Neurological observations including pupil size and reactivity should be carried out and documented prior to departure

- Cervical collars and spinal boards must be used where appropriate, secured appropriately, taking care to avoid jugular venous obstruction
- Use end-tidal CO_2 monitors on all head-injured patients so that CO_2 may be monitored and controlled (and adequate cerebral perfusion pressure may be considered)
- All head injured children should be nursed (where possible) midline with 30° head–up tilt to decrease intracranial pressure
- Intrathoracic and intra-abdominal injuries adequately investigated and appropriately managed
- Long bone/pelvic fractures stabilised
- Raised intracranial pressure appropriately managed
- Seizures controlled
- Measures to maintain blood sugar in normal range if appropriate.

Temperature control

- Measures to maintain normothermia and prevent hyperthermia in situ if appropriate
- Take temperature at referring hospital
- Use mittens, socks, hats, gamgee, blankets, transport incubator, ambulance heater and other available products as appropriate to maintain adequate body temperature, considering the season and length of journey as well as the child's illness.

Drugs/fluids

- Sedation and paralysing drugs infusing/to hand if intubated
- Drugs drawn up for intubation/reintubation
- Normal saline flushes and volume drawn up in syringes sealed with a bung
- All drugs/fluids labelled accurately
- Resuscitation drugs calculated and drawn up, to hand if required
- Appropriate handling, administration and documentation of controlled drugs
- Maintenance fluid if required
- Appropriate storage and use of blood products if required.

Family and communication

- Good introduction to child, family and referring team on arrival
- Talk to family to update on child's condition
- Ensure all essential documentation complete, i.e. names, contact telephone numbers
- Ensure family knows which PICU their child will be taken to and that they have all contact details

- If possible, i.e. if space, insurance and retrieval policy allow, take a parent with team in ambulance – making clear the expectations of the team during the journey (i.e. must remain seated, seatbelt fastened, must allow team to treat child first without distraction in case of emergency)
- Telephone receiving PICU prior to leaving referring hospital to update on child's condition and give estimated time of arrival (also important to let them know about any special requirements, e.g. need for cubicle, need for immediate CVVH therapy or inotrope change on arrival)
- Telephone referring hospital on arrival in PICU to inform them of safe transfer.

Documentation

Transfer details:

- Name, address including post code, date of birth
- Next of kin, names and contact details
- Parents' marital status should be recorded for purposes of consent if further treatment is required
- Name and address of GP
- Referring ward, hospital and telephone number
- Name of referring doctor and contact details
- Receiving doctor, ward, hospital and contact details
- Names and status of escorting personnel in retrieval team.

A medical summary

- Diagnosis and reason for requiring intensive care
- History and past history
- Intubation history, ventilatory support and blood gases
- CVS status including fluid, inotrope and vasopressor requirements
- Medication given
- Intravenous access and monitoring lines
- Recent results and MRSA, RSV, pertussis, etc. status or recent exposure to infectious disease, e.g. chicken pox
- Vaccination history.

A nursing summary

- Observations, documentation of vital signs during transfer
- Drugs and fluids given during transfer
- Respiratory and cardiovascular status, communication method, nutrition, pain and sedation, elimination, skin condition, social and family needs (particularly any child protection issues)
- Summary of patient's condition during transfer.

Audit data

- Severity of illness
- Reason for transfer
- Response times
- Adverse incidents.

IN TRANSIT

- Change from the portable O_2 cylinder to the ambulance supply
- Check that all your emergency equipment and drugs are nearby (on charge if possible) and not moving around the ambulance
- Check that you have a clear view of the child and all the monitors and pumps
- Ask the crew to adjust the temperature of the ambulance according to your needs
- Some teams carry portable blood gas analysers, others find end-tidal CO_2 monitors useful in assessing the child's ventilation requirements
- If the ventilated child is going to be hand-bagged for any reason, you might be able to take turns doing this with the doctor – it can be a tiring job on a long journey!
- Make sure all members of the team and any parents use their seatbelts
- If you need to administer treatment, ask the ambulance crew to slow down/stop
- Record observations, drug dosages, etc. according to your unit policy – commonly this is done every 15 min
- Observe the child and monitors closely for signs of deterioration in vital signs/lightening level of consciousness/fitting
- In the event of an acute deterioration, the ambulance will need to pull over and stop, and you may need to request the help of the crew, e.g. if the child has a cardiac arrest
- In these situations, a call ahead to your unit to inform them of a major problem; this will enable them to assist you immediately on arrival if required.

LOOKING AFTER YOURSELF

Retrievals can involve many hours of travelling and working in hot, stressful conditions. It is a good idea to take cartons of juice and snacks with you, and the referring unit may offer tea or coffee. Some people find nausea a problem, particularly on long journeys in the back of a swaying ambulance. Many of the new ambulances have forward-facing seats, which can help, as can opening the sliding windows a little to let some air in. Some people find sweets helpful and mints are highly rec-ommended! If nausea becomes a real problem on retrieval journeys, you may need to consider trying anti-nausea wrist bands or appropriate medication to relieve it.

Remember to update the referring unit regularly on the condition of the child, particularly shortly after admission and when the child leaves the unit.

Air retrievals have not been discussed here – they carry their own specific problems, whether using a fixed-wing or helicopter service, and staff need to be fully familiar with these.

REFERENCES

Barry PW, Ralston C 1994, Adverse events occurring during interhospital transfer of the critically ill. Arch Dis Childh 71: 8–11

British Paediatric Association 1993 Report of a working party on paediatric intensive care. British Paediatric Association, London

CEN 1999 Medical vehicles and their equipment – Road ambulances. European Standard EN 1789. European Committee for Standardisation, Brussels

Department of Health 1997a Paediatric intensive care: a framework for the future. Department of Health, London

Department of Health 1997b A bridge to the future: nursing standards, education and workforce planning in paediatric intensive care. Department of Health, London

King BR, Woodward GA 2001 Procedural training for pediatric and neonatal transport nurses: Part 1 – Training methods and airway training. Pediatr Emerg Care 17: 461–464

Melville M, Print M 1996 Legal issues surrounding neonatal emergency transport: minimising the risk of litigation. J Neonat Nurs 2: 18–22

Paediatric Intensive Care Society 1996 Standards for paediatric intensive care. Paediatric Intensive Care Society, London

Paediatric Intensive Care Society 2001 Standards document 2001. Paediatric Intensive Care Society, London

UKCC 1992 Scope of professional practice. United Kingdom Central Council for Nursing, Health Visiting and Midwifery, London

FURTHER READING

Davies J 2001 Paediatric retrieval – aiming for the gold standard. Care Crit Ill 17: 94–98

Intensive Care Society 2002 Transport of the critically ill adult. Intensive Care Society Standards. Intensive Care Society, London

Useful website

www.cenorm.be

DEATH OF A CHILD

12

THE NURSE'S ROLE

When a child dies suddenly in hospital, nurses play a central role in caring for the parents and providing essential information. Parents should be offered a private place to hold, cuddle, wash, dress or just to be near their child for as long as they wish and a nurse should be available to support the parents if desired. A private telephone should be made available for their use to contact close family and friends. It is important to refer to local and national policies when caring for a family following the death of a child. Often, when babies or young children die, parents like to have hand and footprints made to treasure and keep. Many parents like to keep a lock of their child's hair but permission should be sought before taking either. If the parents wish, a photograph may be taken of the child, where possible, when all invasive lines and medical equipment have been removed and s/he has been washed and dressed but, again, it is vital that permission is given by the parents. A photograph including the family also may be helpful for the parents to keep. Some parents want the keepsakes at the time, but a few may call after several weeks asking for them, and therefore they must be kept safely. Often a favourite toy, a piece of jewellery, a rosary or a hand-made card from a sibling is left with the child who has died and may be buried with them. It is important to offer the support of a chaplain, priest or spiritual leader according to the needs of the particular family.

In the UK, if a post-mortem is not required, it may be possible for parents to take their child's body home soon after his/her death, if they so wish. A death certificate must have been completed and given to the parents. Nurses must follow local policy, paying particular attention to all documentation (e.g. ensuring that the mortuary paperwork is completed even if the child's body is not actually taken to the mortuary). A small child may be wrapped up in a blanket and transported home in a family member's car. A letter should be given to the parents to take in the car explaining, in case of an accident, that their child died in hospital and that the body is being transported home. Parents should also be given an information sheet about caring for their child's body. Larger children can be taken home with the assistance of a funeral director and, in all cases, early contact with the funeral directors is vital.

It should be noted, however, that there are some infections – e.g. yellow fever, Creutzfeldt–Jakob disease – that require that the child who has died should immediately be placed in a sealed coffin. The sealed coffin can be taken to the parents' home if they so wish. (For full list of infections see Appendix 6, Paediatric Intensive Care Society 2002.)

It is very important that relevant people have been informed of the child's death as soon as possible so that appropriate care may be given by

---

Box 12.1 Standards for bereavement care

Care of the family
- See the family as the unit of care
- Give them time
- Make parents aware of any choices and seek parents' views
- Respect their cultural, spiritual and religious needs
- Help them to include siblings.

Prior to death
- Involve parents in any decision to withdraw care
- Explain what may happen
- Explain possibility of taking child home
- Multidisciplinary team approach.

Brain stem death tests
If brain stem testing is to be carried out, give parents an explanation of what may happen, explain probable findings and ask parents if they wish to be present.

Organ donation
If relevant, a collaborative approach is recommended; discuss this as fully as possible with a doctor trained in obtaining consent for organ donation, the donor transplant coordinator and the bedside nurse. Ideally, there should be two nurses on duty at any time who have been trained in the principles of organ donation.
  Parents should be given written information, including:

- Detail of possible coroner involvement and post-mortem
- When and where to collect the death certificate
- How to register the child's death
- Who to contact to arrange a funeral and information regarding the social fund, if paying for the child's funeral may pose a problem
- Addresses of support groups, information regarding books, videos, etc.
- An invitation for the family to come back to see the consultant if they wish to discuss any unanswered issues
- The name of a known professional worker who cared for the child and family whom they can contact at work if they need any other information or help.

Source: Paediatric Intensive Care Society 2002

all agencies, e.g. GP, health visitor, school, social worker and referring hospital. The specialist nurses/bereavement worker, e.g. a family support sister, if in post, should be informed of each child's death and given all the relevant details and particular circumstances so that they can maintain contact with the family and provide follow-up care. Many children's hospitals have a 'Ronald MacDonald House' or similar home where parents stay while their child is in hospital and they should also be informed of a child's death.

BRAIN STEM DEATH

The Department of Health set up a Working Party in 1998 that devised *A Code of Practice for the Diagnosis of Brain Stem Death*; their definition of death is: 'irreversible loss of capacity for consciousness, combined with irreversible loss of the capacity to breathe'. Brain stem death may occur before cardiorespiratory function ceases. It is important that nurses understand and can explain the concept of brain stem death. Brain stem death tests are usually carried out by the consultant in charge of the child's care and one other clinically independent doctor, competent in the field and not a member of the transplant team, who has been qualified for at least 5 years. The tests are performed twice and, prior to testing, time must have elapsed to ensure that the patient has no circulating or therapeutic levels of any drug that could cause coma. A diagnosis must have been established and the cause of the coma must be irreversible. Prior to testing, the child should be normothermic, with no endocrine or metabolic disturbances, and have no effects of muscle relaxants in his/her system.

The British Paediatric Association (Conference of Medical Royal Colleges and their Faculties in the UK 1991) guidelines for paediatric brain stem testing recommend that the child should be a minimum age of 37 weeks gestation plus 2 months, as it is rarely possible to confidently diagnose brain stem death between the ages of 37 weeks gestation and 2 months of age. Below the age of 37 weeks gestation the criteria for brain stem death cannot be applied.

Clinical tests for brain stem death

- Pupils are fixed and dilated and do not react to light
- Absent corneal reflexes – tested by touching exposed cornea with a piece of cotton wool but take care to avoid damage
- Absent oculovestibular reflexes – ice cold water is syringed into each ear in turn, having ensured that the passage to the tympanic membrane is clear. Normally this would produce eye movement, where there is deviation to the stimulated side
- No cranial nerve motor response to deep, painful stimulation within the cranial nerve distribution
- Absent cough or gag reflex – this is tested with deep suction via the endotracheal tube and to the back of the throat

- Apnoea test – the partial pressure of carbon dioxide (P_aCO_2) should be 5.3 kPa (40 mmHg) prior to the apnoea test and should rise to at least 6.6 kPa (50 mmHg) during the test if the patient remains apnoeic. The patient should be preoxygenated with 100% oxygen for 10 min prior to testing and arterial blood gases should be taken. The patient is disconnected from the ventilator but given a continuous supply of 100% oxygen via the endotracheal tube. The patient is observed for 10 min to note any respiratory effort and then another arterial blood gas is taken to ensure that the P_aCO_2 has risen above 6.6 kPa (50 mmHg). The patient is then reconnected to the ventilator. This test must be discontinued if hypotension, cardiac arrhythmias or hypoxia occurs.

If the first test shows brain stem death, the legal time of death is recorded on completion of this first set of brain stem tests and must be declared in the medical notes. Death is not pronounced until the second set of tests has been completed.

Spinal reflexes: the spinal cord may continue to function after the death of the brain stem, and the resulting limb movement may be distressing to the family and staff caring for the patient. Nurses should be aware of this potential occurrence and be able to give the family an explanation.

If appropriate, the opportunity for organ donation must be offered to families once brain stem death has been established.

THE PROCESS OF ORGAN DONATION

Consider making the transplant co-ordinators aware of the potential organ donor prior to brain stem testing so that a collaborative approach can be taken when talking to the family about organ donation. When a child is found to be brain stem dead, the family is offered the opportunity to donate their child's organs. The family will need time and privacy to discuss the matter. The donor transplant coordinator will come to the unit to discuss all aspects with the family. If the family still wish to continue, full explanations should be given at this time about the likelihood of needing to continue treatment to maintain the organs in the best possible condition. It must be consistently reinforced that the child is brain stem dead and that no treatment can change that. Consent will then be obtained if the family wish to proceed with the donation of their child's organs.

Once recipients have been found for the organs, a team of surgeons will come to retrieve the organs. Major organs will not be removed unless a matched recipient has been identified. The donor's family will usually say their goodbyes at this time, then the child is taken to theatre with cardiopulmonary function being maintained and supported.

Once the organs have been retrieved, they are taken, swiftly, to be transplanted into the recipients. The donor child's body will be carefully sutured and then taken to the mortuary or back to the ward if the parents wish to spend more time saying their goodbyes. The time taken between parents deciding to donate their child's organs and the time the child is actually taken to theatre is usually less than 12 hours, and parents have the right to change their mind at any time. The process described is concerned with solid organ donation, as some tissues, e.g. heart valves and corneas, may be retrieved the following day.

NB The parents may wish to come back to see their child in the hospital chapel following donation of their child's organs, and they may wish to hold and cuddle their child, so it may be advisable to gently inform them that:

- their child will feel cold to the touch
- their child will look very pale
- their child will have a suture line where the organs have been removed but this will be covered with a dressing
- their child may feel lighter in weight if they pick him/her up for a cuddle
- their child's abdomen may appear flatter or concave if large organs have been donated.

MULTIORGAN DONATION

Age criteria

(These are approximate as all potential donors are assessed individually.)

- **Kidneys** 2–75 years (paediatric donors are assessed according to size and weight)
- **Liver** 0–70 years
- **Heart** 0–60 years (if unsuitable, the heart valves may be considered)
- **Lungs** 0–60 years
- **Pancreas** 18–45 years (outside these age limits, the pancreas may be donated for research).

Other criteria

- Age, as previously described, according to the British Paediatric Association guidelines
- A confirmed diagnosis of brain stem death
- Artificially ventilated
- No past medical or social history contraindications – no current or past history of malignancy, except for tissue-diagnosed primary brain tumour and not categorised high-risk
- Coroner's consent
- Consent from legal next of kin
- Virology screen (negative HIV and hepatitis B and C).

Multiorgan donors may also donate tissues

- Corneas 6 months–100 years (poor eyesight is not a contraindication)
- Heart valves 6 months–60 years.

(Trachea and skin may also be donated, but not from paediatric patients.)

INVESTIGATIONS THAT MAY BE REQUIRED PRIOR TO ORGAN DONATION

This is the responsibility of the transplant co-ordinator but it requires team work and it may be helpful to liaise with the coordinator and to begin to obtain the necessary tests so that the process takes as little time as possible.

- Virology screen – 10 ml of blood in plain blood tube (it may be necessary to take a virology screen from the mother if the child is under 2 years of age)
- Blood group and tissue type
- Urea and electrolytes
- Liver function tests
- Arterial blood gases
- Clotting studies
- Sputum Gram stain
- Chest X-ray
- Electrocardiogram
- Amylase
- Echocardiogram
- Culture and sensitivity screens – wounds, sputum, urine.

CLINICAL MANAGEMENT GUIDELINES OF THE ORGAN DONOR

(Reproduced with permission from Marchant 1997.)

Common clinical problems that may occur in a brain stem dead patient include:

- Hypotension
- Hypothermia
- Endocrine disturbances
- Electrolyte imbalance
- Arrhythmias
- Hypoxia
- Coagulopathy
- Neurogenic pulmonary oedema.

Hypotension

Causes Loss of vasomotor tone, myocardial depression, hypovolaemia due to blood loss, diuretics, vasodilation or diabetes insipidus.

Effect Poor organ perfusion with potential ischaemia.

Management Filling, preferably with colloid solution, inotropes – dobutamine, dopamine and adrenaline (epinephrine) – as a last resort.

Goal Normotension, central venous pressure (CVP) 5–10 cmH$_2$O, urine output 1 mL/kg/min.

Hypothermia

Causes Loss of temperature regulation and vasomotor tone aggravated by hypovolaemia.

Effect Risk of arrhythmias, decreased basal metabolic rate, increased oxidisers.

Management Warm slowly using warming blanket, warm IV fluids, warm inhaled gases.

Goal Temperature 35–37°C.

Endocrine disturbances – diabetes insipidus

Causes Cerebral ischaemia, raised intracranial pressure, hypoxia.

Effect Polyuria causing gross hypovolaemia, electrolyte imbalance.

Management Do not fluid-deplete, **do not stop dopamine**, investigate fluid replacement therapy, administer DDAVP but avoid giving this within 2 h of going to theatre.

Goal Normalise urine output and concentration.

Electrolyte imbalance

Common electrolyte disturbances experienced are hypokalaemia, hypocalcaemia and hypernatraemia.

Causes Blood loss, diabetes insipidus, inadequate replacement therapy.

Effect Cardiac arrhythmia, poor cardiac contractility, asystole.

Management Monitor and correct imbalance.

Goal Normal values.

Hypoxia

Causes Trauma, aspiration, sputum retention, pulmonary oedema.

Effect Poor tissue and organ perfusion.

Management Physiotherapy, including bagging and suction, frequent turning, bronchoscopy, correct CO_2 and frequent ABG, avoid excessive crystalloid infusion, add PEEP.

Goal $P_aO_2 > 11.0\,kPa$ ($>83\,mmHg$), airway pressures $<30\,cmH_2O$, clear chest X-ray, $F_iO_2 < 0.4$, audible clear air entry.

Coagulopathy

Causes The ischaemic brain and resultant catecholamine storm releases fibrinolytic agents into the circulation.

Effect Presentation of a disseminated intravascular coagulation (DIC)-type picture.

Management Administration of relevant clotting factors, monitor clotting studies, observe for clinical signs of haemorrhage, rule out possibility of underlying, undiagnosed haematological disorder.

Neurogenic pulmonary oedema

Causes Catecholamine surge in response to intracranial insult may cause a sudden increase in systemic vascular resistance, with a shift of blood flow from the systemic circulation to the pulmonary circulation.

Effect Hypoxia leading to poor tissue and organ perfusion.

Management Assess fluid status, redo chest X-ray, consider reversing I:E ratio, add PEEP, continue to monitor blood gases, continue physiotherapy, **do not give up**.

Goal Normalised arterial blood gases with no pulmonary oedema. If management is unsuccessful, the lungs may be unsuitable for donation.

RELIGION

There are no religious denominations that object to organ or tissue donation; however, it is advisable to be aware of individual requirements for the care of the deceased. It may be important for the next of kin to liaise with their religious leader regarding donation. This is always respected.

REFERENCES

Conference of Medical Royal Colleges and their Faculties in the UK 1991 Diagnosis of brainstem death in infants and children. British Paediatric Association, London

Department of Health 1998 A code of practice for the diagnosis of brain stem death: including guidelines for the identification and management of potential organ and tissue donors. HMSO, London

Paediatric Intensive Care Society 2002 Standards for bereavement care. Paediatric Intensive Care Society, London

FURTHER READING

Human Tissue Act 1961 HMSO, London

Marchant C 1997 The organ donation information folder. South Thames Transplant Co-ordination Service, London

CHILD DEVELOPMENT

13

It is useful for nurses to have some knowledge of normal child development in order to be able to assess a child thoroughly on admission. Each child is different and the parents/carers may be the best source of information about developmental milestones achieved. It has been shown that some children regress developmentally when they are admitted to hospital or in other stressful circumstances. This chapter is intended as a guide to normal child development.

STAGES OF COGNITIVE DEVELOPMENT (PIAGET & INHELDER 1969)

- 0–2 years: sensorimotor stage
- 2–6 years: preoperational stage
- 6–12 years: concrete operational stage
- 12 years+: formal operational stage.

Sensorimotor stage

The infant's response to the world is almost entirely sensory and motor. This stage may be subdivided into six substages:

- 0–1 month: reflexes (Box 13.1)
- 1–4 months: primary circular reactions (e.g. putting finger into mouth)

Box 13.1   Seven major reflexes in the newborn

- **Rooting**: infant will turn towards the touch of a cheek, searching for something to suck
- **Sucking**: sucking results from putting something into the infant's mouth
- **Swallowing**: initially not well coordinated with breathing
- **Moro**: when startled, infants will arch their backs and throw open their arms
- **Grasp**: infants will curl their fingers around any object that can be grasped
- **Babinski**: if an infant is stroked on the bottom of the foot, the toes splay out, then curl in
- **Stepping**: if infants are held so that their feet just touch the ground, they will initiate walking movements

Source: from Bee 1989

- 4–10 months: secondary circular reactions (i.e. beginning to realise that own actions have external results)
- 10 months–1 year: coordination of secondary schemes (i.e. combining actions to achieve a result)
- 1–1.5 years: tertiary circular actions (improving motor skills)
- 1.5–2 years: beginning of thought.

Preoperational stage

This stage involves the use of images, words or actions that convey something else, e.g. pretend play. Initially children in this stage are egocentric – they see the world only in their own perspective – but this view widens during this stage as the child learns to share.

Concrete operational stage

During this stage logic and reasoning develop. The child begins to understand the concept of reversibility and the principles of conservation.

Formal operational stage

During this stage the child develops deductive reasoning and a systematic problem-solving approach.

FREUD'S STAGES OF PSYCHOSEXUAL DEVELOPMENT

Freud (1964) looked differently at child development, as shown in Table 13.1.

NORMAL CHILD DEVELOPMENT – WHAT TO EXPECT OF A CHILD OF A CERTAIN AGE (WHALEY & WONG 1991, ENGEL 1993)

Newborn

- Reflexes as previously described
- Normal range of cries, including differing cries for hunger or pain

Table 13.1 Freud's stages of psychosexual development

Age	Stage	Developmental task
0–1 year	Oral	Weaning
2–3 years	Anal	Toilet training
4–5 years	Phallic	Identification with parent of same sex
6–12 years	Latency	Development of ego
13–18 years	Genital	Mature sexual intimacy

- Vision: best able to focus eyes at a distance of 25 cm
- Unable to hold head up but can turn head to side when prone
- Hands held with fingers curled into a fist.

Six weeks

- Starts to smile
- Starts to coo in response to the sound of mother's voice
- Developing head control.

Three months

- Starts laughing
- Can hold head up beyond the plane of the rest of the body
- Has only slight head lag when pulled to sit
- Follows an object for 180° when lying supine
- Turns head to sound
- Posterior fontanelle now closed.

Six months

- No head lag when pulled to sit
- Sits without support
- Starts babbling
- Teething begins
- Can chew on soft food
- Can transfer object from one hand to another
- Increasing fear of strangers.

Nine months

- Pulls to a standing position
- Crawls on tummy
- Babbles repetitive syllables
- Can pick up a small object between thumb and forefinger.

One year

- Walks with one hand held
- Knows own name
- Can speak 2–3 words clearly
- Can drink from cup with help
- Begins casting objects
- Clings to mother when in unfamiliar situations.

Eighteen months

- Begins to identify objects
- Vocabulary around 50 words
- Begins to combine two words as a sentence
- Points to object and can feed self
- Jumps using both feet
- Can build a tower of 3–4 cubes
- Begins to scribble
- Anterior fontanelle closes
- Can use a spoon but will turn it upside down before it reaches the mouth.

Two years

- Talks to self during play
- Vocabulary around 300 words
- Knows 4 body parts
- Can put on pants, socks and shoes
- Mainly dry at night.

Four years

- Has conversational speech
- Can write own name
- Can count
- Vocabulary of around 1500 words
- Can dress and undress
- Enjoys imaginary play.

Six years

- Vocabulary of several thousand words
- Increasing dexterity, can run, jump and ride a bike
- Knows right from left
- May show jealousy of siblings
- Enjoys playing games.

Eight years

- Increasing manual dexterity, can use most household utensils
- Learns principles of conversation
- Keen to be involved in clubs, likes company of others
- Able to classify
- Can count backwards from 20
- Likes to help.

Ten years

- Height slowly increasing
- Weight increasing rapidly
- Start of puberty for some children
- Has logical thinking
- Best friends are important
- Can wash and dry own hair
- May begin to show interest in the opposite sex.

Adolescence

- Increasing weight and height
- Girls may commence menstruation
- Bodily changes associated with puberty
- Mood swings
- Conflicts with parents
- Increasing capacity for abstract reasoning
- Developing sexual identity.

CHILDREN'S DEVELOPMENTAL CONCEPTS OF PAIN

It is important that nurses understand children's cognitive development and their perceptions of pain at each developmental stage.

Hurley & Whelan (1988) describe children's concepts of pain according to Piaget's cognitive developmental stages. The sensorimotor stage is omitted as these children are unable to vocalise their perceptions of pain.

Preoperational stage (2–7 years)

- These children may think that pain is a punishment for something that they have done wrong
- They may blame someone else for their pain
- They relate to pain primarily as a physical experience
- They often have feelings of sadness when in pain so may feel comforted if held and given reassurance.

Concrete operational stage (7–10 years)

- These children can understand physical pain and can locate the pain to the relevant part of the body
- They fear bodily harm and death
- They like to feel they have some control over the pain so they should be encouraged to ask for help to find the most comfortable position or to ask for pain relief.

Table 13.2 General features of common childhood illnesses

Disease	Type	Spread	Signs/symptoms	Incubation	Contagious
Measles	Viral	Coughs/sneezes	Fever, runny nose, cough, then rash after few days	10–12 days after exposure	4 d before rash to about 4 d after
Mumps	Viral	Direct contact with saliva or discharge from nose/throat	Fever, swelling and tenderness of salivary glands (sometimes orchiditis in boys)	Usually 16–18 d after exposure	3 d before and up to 4 d after onset of symptoms
Rubella	Rubella virus	Close contact with coughs and sneezes	Usually mild disease – slight fever, rash on face and neck for 2–3 d	12–23 d after exposure	1 week before rash to 1 week after rash, but most contagious while rash visible
Chicken pox	Varicella–zoster virus	Through air by coughs and sneezes or by direct contact with fluid from blisters	Fever, itchy rash all over body – fluid-filled vesicles	14–21 d after exposure	1–2 d before rash appears until all blisters have dried up (usually 4–5 d)
Pertussis	*Bordetella pertussis* bacterial infection	Personal contact, coughs, sneezes	Cold, sneezes, fever, cough then after 1 week cough becomes severe and can last for 6 weeks	7–10 d from exposure	1 week from exposure until up to 3 weeks after the severe cough starts

Formal operational stage (12 years +)

- These children are able to use reasoning, e.g. my head hurts because I banged it.
- They fear loss of privacy and control when in pain
- They need to be given as much information as they require and choices about how best to control the pain.

IMMUNISATION SCHEDULE

When taking a history from parents about their child's development and health it is important to establish whether the child has been immunised fully. The current immunisation schedule is included so that health-care professionals can check if all the correct immunisations have been given. Of course immunisation schedules sometimes change, but website addresses are given at the end of this chapter so that up to date information can always be obtained.

Summary of immunisation schedule 0–5 years (Department of Health 2006)

DTaP/IPV/Hib is a single vaccine that protects against diphtheria, tetanus, pertussis, polio and Hib. In February 2006 the pneumococcal vaccine was introduced into the immunisation schedule, the three doses of meningitis C were respaced (from vaccine at 2, 3 and 4 months to vaccine at 3, 4 and booster at 12 months) and a booster of Hib was added at 12 months (Department of Health 2006/0056)

- At 2 months DTaP/IPV/Hib + pneumococcal vaccine
- 3 months DTaP/IPV/Hib + meningitis C vaccine
- 4 months DTaP/IPV/Hib + meningitis C + pneumococcal vaccine
- 12 months Hib + meningitis C
- 13 months Measles, mumps and rubella (MMR) + pneumococcal vaccine
- 3–5 years (preschool) DTaP/IPV/Hib + MMR.

See Table 13.2 for general features of common childhood illnesses.

REFERENCES

Bee H 1989 The developing child, 5th edn. Harper & Row, New York
Department of Health 2004 New vaccinations for the childhood immunisation programme. Department of Health, London
Engel J 1993 Pocket guide pediatric assessment, 2nd edn. CV Mosby, St Louis, MO

Freud S 1964 An outline of psychoanalysis. Hogarth Press, London

Hurley A, Whelan EG 1988 Cognitive development and children's perception of pain. Pediatr Nurs 14: 21–24

Piaget J, Inhelder B 1969 The psychology of the child. Routledge & Kegan Paul, London

Whaley LF, Wong DL 1991 Nursing care of infants and children, 4th edn. CV Mosby, St Louis, MO

FURTHER READING

Illingworth RS 1993 The normal child, 10th edn. Churchill Livingstone, Edinburgh

Sylva K, Lunt I 1990 Child development: a first course. Blackwell, Oxford

CHILD PROTECTION

14

All those who come into contact with children and families in their everyday work, including practitioners who do not have a specific role in relation to safeguarding children, have a duty to safeguard and promote the welfare of children.

THE NURSE'S INVOLVEMENT

You are likely to be involved in three main ways:

- You may have concerns about a child, and refer those concerns to children's social care or the police
- You may be approached by children's social care and asked to provide information about a child or family, or to be involved in an assessment. This may happen regardless of who made the referral to children's social care
- You may be asked to provide help or a specific service to the child or family as part of an agreed plan and contribute to the reviewing of the child's progress (Department for Education and Skills 2006).

POTENTIAL GROUNDS FOR CONCERN

You may suspect that a child is being abused if you have any concerns about the following:

- Health and development
- General appearance
- Behaviour
- Parent and child relationship
- Unexplained injuries
- Inappropriate explanation for injuries
- A chance 'trigger' remark
- Information from a third party
- Problems in the carer's home, e.g. domestic violence, alcohol or drug abuse.

PROCESSES FOR SAFEGUARDING CHILDREN

The following flow charts illustrate the processes for safeguarding children:

1. From the point that concerns are raised and are referred to a statutory agency that can take action to safeguard and promote the welfare of the child (Fig. 14.1)
2. Through an initial assessment of the child's situation and what happens after that (Fig. 14.2)

Fig. 14.1 Referral (with permission from Department for Education and Skills 2006)

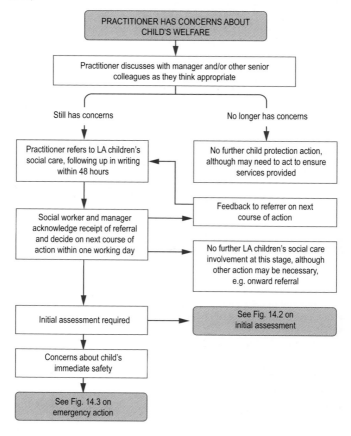

3. Taking urgent action, if necessary (Fig. 14.3)
4. To the strategy discussion, where there are concerns about the child's safety, and beyond that to the child protection conference (Fig. 14.4)

Fig. 14.2 What happens following initial assessment? (with permission from Department for Education and Skills 2006)

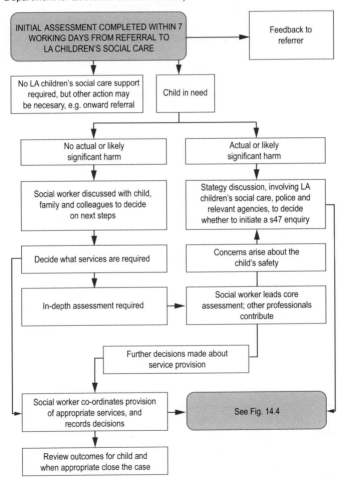

Fig. 14.3 Urgent action to safeguard children (with permission from Department for Education and Skills 2006)

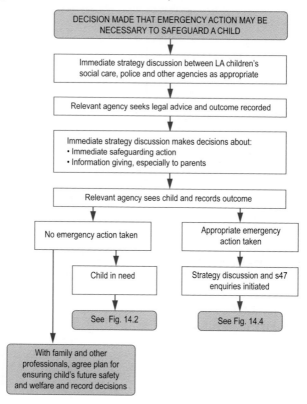

5. What happens after the child protection conference, and the review process (Fig. 14.5).

 A number of the many recommendations from Lord Laming's report (Department of Health 2003) relate to ensuring effective communication — including accurate and thorough documentation — takes place between health professionals. This includes the need to work from a single set of records for each child.

Fig. 14.4 What happens after the strategy discussion? (with permission from Department for Education and Skills 2006)

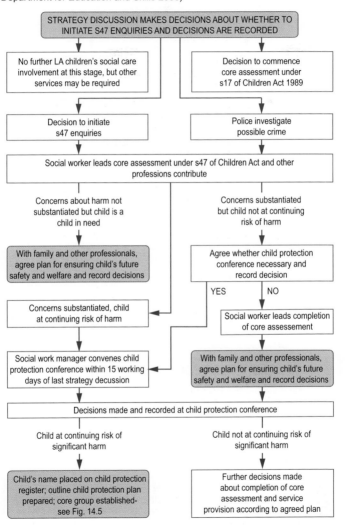

Fig. 14.5   What happens after the child protection conference, including the review process? (with permission from Department for Education and Skills 2006)

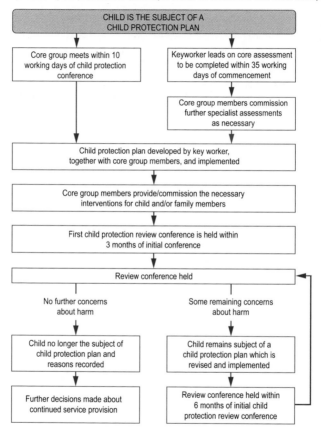

REFERENCES

Department for Education and Skills 2006 What to do if you are worried a child is being abused – Summary. Department for Education and Skills, Nottingham. Available on line at: www.everychildmatters.gov.uk/resources-and-practice/IG00182

Department of Health 2003 The Victoria Climbié enquiry: report of an enquiry by Lord Laming. Department of Health, London

FURTHER READING

Department for Education and Skills 2005 The Children Act 2004.
Available on line at: www.dfes.gov.uk/publications/childrenactreport/

Department of Health 2004 National Service Framework for children,
young people and maternity services. Stationery Office, London

Framework for the Assessment of Children in Need and their Families.
Available on line at: www.doh.gov.uk

Working Together to Safeguard Children: a guide to interagency working
to safeguard and promote the welfare of children. Available on line at:
www.doh.gov.uk

Infants and children may present in A&E or a PICU with a collection of unexplained symptoms and signs that may lead to diagnosis of a previously undiagnosed syndrome. The following list is not comprehensive but provides a quick reference to the more common syndromes.

The term 'congenital' means existing at and usually before birth. At the end of the chapter are a few website addresses that can provide invaluable information for medical staff and families.

CHROMOSOMAL DISORDERS

There may be addition or deletion of chromosomes.

Cri du chat syndrome

This syndrome occurs as a result of partial deletion of the short arm of chromosome 5. A characteristic of this syndrome is a high-pitched cry, which resembles the 'cry' of a cat.

Appearance: Craniofacial abnormalities, microcephaly and a moon-shaped face with hypertelorism (increased interpupillary distance).

These children have severe learning difficulties and an increased incidence of congenital heart defects.

DiGeorge's syndrome

This syndrome is usually a sporadic malformation but some patients show a microdeletion of chromosome 22. The thymus and parathyroid glands are absent because of defective development of the third and fourth embryonic pharyngeal pouches. This is characterised by neonatal tetany, hypocalcaemia and frequent viral infections.

Appearance: Dysmorphic features.
There may be aortic arch anomalies.

Down's syndrome (trisomy 21)

An extra chromosome 21 characterises the best recognised chromosome disorder.

Appearance: Small, slanting eyes, low-set ears, prominent epicanthic (neck) folds, small mouth causing frequent tongue protrusion and commonly there is a single transverse palmar crease.

These children will have learning difficulties with a reduced IQ. Down's syndrome is often associated with a congenital heart lesion, umbilical hernia, higher than normal incidence of duodenal atresia, Hirschsprung's disease and leukaemia.

Edwards' syndrome (trisomy 18)

Appearance: The baby will have protruding eyes, low-set malformed ears, a receding chin, flexion deformities of the hands with the index finger overlapping the third digit, and characteristic feet with a prominent heel and convex sole ('rocker-bottom feet'). Infants usually have major cardiac anomalies and survival is uncommon beyond 6 months.

Klinefelter's syndrome (XXY)

This syndrome affects males only and means that their chromosome pattern is XXY and they are infertile. It is often undiagnosed until adolescence.

Appearance: Tall in stature with unusually long legs, hypogonadism and gynaecomastia. There is increased incidence of learning difficulties.

Prader–Willi syndrome

In approximately 50% of patients with this syndrome there is a small deletion in the long arm on chromosome 15 (Connor & Ferguson-Smith 1987).

Appearance: Round face with a prominent forehead and a pronounced nasal bridge, short stature, small hands and feet, obesity and hypogonadism.

These children are initially hypotonic and have delayed motor development, feeding difficulties and learning difficulties.

Turner's syndrome (X0)

This syndrome affects females only. They have only 45 chromosomes and have a chromosome pattern of X0.

Appearance: Short stature, micrognathia (small jaw), webbing of the neck, lymphoedema, widely spaced nipples, failure to develop breasts.

Normal lifespan and intelligence but increased incidence of congenital heart defects, particularly coarctation of the aorta and atrial septal defect. Most females with Turner's syndrome are infertile.

MUCOPOLYSACCHARIDOSES

There are four main types:

Type 1 – Hurler's syndrome

This is a sex-linked recessive trait that affects only males. It results from a deficiency of the enzyme α-L-iduronidase.

Appearance: Abnormal facial features, an enlarged tongue, clouded corneas, short neck and trunk, joint deformities and angular kyphosis.

Hepatosplenomegaly, deafness and cardiac defects are common and the children will have learning difficulties. Large quantities of dermatan sulphate are present in the urine.

Type 2 – Hunter's syndrome

This syndrome is also an autosomal recessive trait that affects only males. The symptoms in Hunter's syndrome are generally milder than those in Hurler's syndrome.

Appearance: Some facial abnormalities but in a milder form than in type 1, angular kyphosis, nodular skin lesions but generally no clouding of the corneas.

These children may also have retinitis pigmentosa, optic atrophy, progressive deafness and pulmonary hypertension. Large quantities of dermatan or heparin sulphate may be present in the urine.

Type 3 – Sanfilippo's syndrome

This syndrome has autosomal recessive inheritance. There is a deficiency of either heparin sulphate sulphamidase or N-acetyl-α -D-glucosaminidase. These children have severe progressive learning difficulties but normal features, no corneal clouding and no cardiac defects.

Type 4 – Morquio's syndrome

This is a rare form of mucopolysaccharidosis that again is an autosomal recessive trait.

Appearance: Short stature, short neck, prominent sternum, scoliosis, waddling gait, protruding mandible and short nose.

These children have normal intelligence but may have mild deafness, clouding of the cornea and perhaps aortic valve disease.

CONGENITAL MALFORMATIONS AND DYSMORPHIC SYNDROMES

The CHARGE and VATER association of symptoms are included in this section.

CHARGE association

CHARGE is an acronym of congenital defects that can occur together:

- C   Coloboma – this is a malformation that results in a cleft in one of the structures of the eye, most commonly the iris
- H   Heart defects
- A   Choanal atresia
- R   Retarded growth and development
- G   Genital hypoplasia
- E   Ear anomalies/deafness.

Children with CHARGE association may also have renal anomalies, tracheo-oesophageal fistula and orofacial problems (Contact-a-Family 1996).

Noonan's syndrome

This is an autosomal dominant trait that affects both sexes but is sometimes known as male Turner's syndrome.

Appearance: Downwards slanting eyes, low-set ears, webbed neck and short stature.
    Learning difficulties and congenital heart defects (most commonly hypertrophic cardiomyopathy or pulmonary stenosis) are often present.

Pierre Robin's syndrome

In this syndrome there is underdevelopment of the lower jaw, micrognathia and glossoptosis (downwards displacement of the tongue), often associated with cleft palate and absent gag reflex. Infants should be nursed on their sides or prone as the tongue is at risk of occluding the airway.

Sturge–Weber syndrome

This is a congenital syndrome that affects the brain, skin and eyes.

Appearance: Facial haemangioma (port-wine stain).
    Intracranial haemangioma is associated with the facial haemangioma. Focal seizures, learning difficulties and glaucoma may occur.

Treacher Collins' syndrome (mandibulofacial dysostosis)

This is an autosomal dominant trait.

Appearance: Characteristic facial appearance – sloping downwards eyes, flat cheeks, hypoplastic mandible, receding chin, large mouth, high palate, low-set ears and deficient cartilage, sometimes with no auditory meatus.

VATER association

This is an acronym for a combination of malformations:
- V   Vertebral defects
- A   Anal atresia
- TE Tracheo–oEsophageal fistula
- R   Renal defects, radial limb dysplasia.

These children have normal intelligence but may also have congenital heart disease.

Wolff–Parkinson–White syndrome

This is a tachydysrhythmia. Cardiac electrical impulses are transmitted along an accessory pathway and therefore atrial impulses can bypass the normal delay that usually occurs at the atrioventricular node. This leads to a rapid re-entry SVT and a characteristic ECG trace with a short P–R interval and a wide QRS interval.

REFERENCES

Connor JM, Ferguson-Smith MA 1987 Essential medical genetics, 2nd edn. Blackwell, Oxford

Contact-a-Family 1996 Directory of specific conditions and rare syndromes in children and their family support networks, 3rd edn. Contact-a-Family, London

FURTHER READING

Hull D, Johnston DI 1985 Essential paediatrics. Churchill Livingstone, Edinburgh

Jolly H, Levene MI 1985 Diseases of children, 5th edn. Blackwell, Oxford

Whaley LF, Wong DL 1991 Nursing care of infants and children, 4th edn. CV Mosby, St Louis, MO

Useful websites

www.happychild.org.uk/syndromes/ – a directory of organisations helping children; information is available in 14 different languages

www.cafamily.org.uk – Contact a Family is a UK-wide charity providing support, advice and information for families with children with special needs. There is a directory of specific conditions and rare disorders.

INDEX

Paediatric basic life support – health-care professionals ith a duty to respond (with permission from Resuscitation Council (UK) 2005)

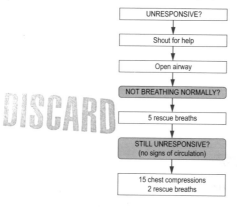

After 1 minute call resuscitation team then continue CPR.

Paediatric advanced life support (with permission from Resuscitation Council (UK) 2005)

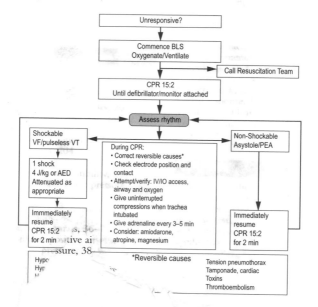